Education Scholarship in Healthcare

April S. Fitzgerald • Gundula Bosch

Editors

Education Scholarship in Healthcare

The Health Scholar's Toolbox

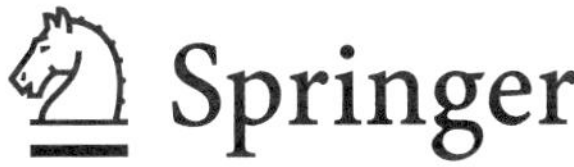 Springer

Editors
April S. Fitzgerald
Johns Hopkins University School
of Medicine
Baltimore, MD, USA

Gundula Bosch
Johns Hopkins Bloomberg School
of Public Health
Baltimore, MD, USA

ISBN 978-3-031-38533-9   ISBN 978-3-031-38534-6   (eBook)
https://doi.org/10.1007/978-3-031-38534-6

This Springer imprint is published by the registered company Springer Nature Switzerland AG
The registered company address is: Gewerbestrasse 11, 6330 Cham, Switzerland

Paper in this product is recyclable.

Introduction

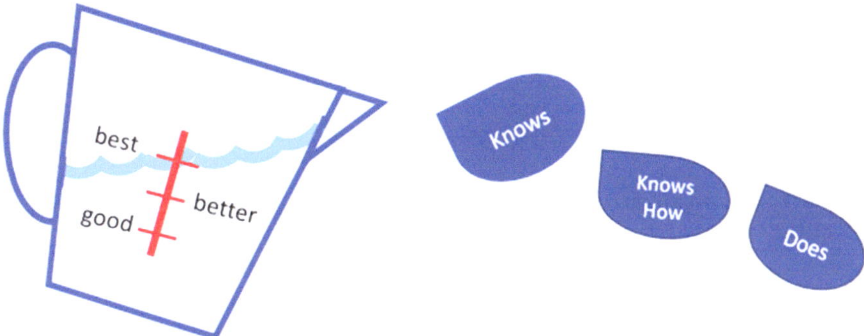

When I arrived at my first academic position, access to the information in this book would have been invaluable, but there was no available resource. It took years of faculty development courses, mentoring, and a Master of Education to accumulate this knowledge. Wanting to help others find an easier path is the genesis for writing this book.

I remember one of my elementary teachers telling our class that she wished for a magic potion. *"The potion,"* she said, *"would effortlessly give you all of the knowledge in the learning plan for this year."*

I imagined my teacher walking down the aisles between our desks, stopping at each student, and administering something mysterious from a measuring cup. At the time, I only considered the student's perspective; we could play games outside at recess all day long!

"Unfortunately," she told us, *"learning doesn't work that way."* She then explained the hard work we would need to invest.

In hindsight, I see my teacher's perspective. She likely desired an innovation to make teaching easier as much as we desired an innovation to make learning easier. That year proved to be memorable for our class. She possessed the educator power to have a lasting impact on our lives.

As an educator in the health profession, you have the power to create impact and change lives. Your talent might be in content creation, instructional design, or noticing a pattern in the system that others overlooked. Educational scholarship amplifies your power through dissemination.

The educational scholarship journey is one of personal growth as you engage with an intellectual academic community and improve your prospects for advancement. The route is a gateway to tremendous opportunity—the creation of new knowledge, the advancement of educational practices, and the ability to shape the field of medicine and the future of healthcare.

Some of you might already have mentors who guide you and answer questions about the pathway ahead—kudos to you. Others might not know whom to ask for help; you are not alone. Whatever your situation, do not worry, because this book gives you both a source of navigation and power. In the chapters, you will find the information and tools to be successful as we journey together.

We are all part of the same team now. We are delighted to have you here. Let us learn and grow together.

Welcome!

April

Contents

Contributors

Sawsan Abdel-Razig, MD, MEHP Department of Medicine, Cleveland Clinic Abu Dhabi, Abu Dhabi, United Arab Emirates

Michael F. Amendola, MD, MEHP Division of Vascular Surgery, Virginia Commonwealth University, Richmond, VA, USA

Anne E. Belcher, PhD, RN Johns Hopkins University School of Education, Baltimore, MD, USA

Gundula Bosch, PhD, MEHP R3 Center for Innovation in Science Education, Department of Molecular Microbiology and Immunology, Johns Hopkins Bloomberg School of Public Health, Baltimore, MD, USA

Camille L. Bryant, PhD, MEd Johns Hopkins University School of Education, Baltimore, MD, USA

April S. Fitzgerald, MD, MEHP Division of General Internal Medicine, Department of Medicine, Johns Hopkins University School of Medicine, Baltimore, MD, USA

Ahmed Ibrahim, PhD, MSc Johns Hopkins University School of Education, Baltimore, MD, USA

Halah Ibrahim, MD, MEHP Department of Medicine, Khalifa University College of Medicine and Health Sciences, Abu Dhabi, UAE

Emily L. Jones, EdD, MEd Johns Hopkins University School of Education, Baltimore, MD, USA

David E. Kern, MD, MPH Johns Hopkins University School of Medicine, Baltimore, MD, USA

Daphne H. Knicely, MD, MEHP Division of Nephrology, Department of Medicine, University of Virginia School of Medicine, Charlottesville, VA, USA

Khanh-Van Le-Bucklin, MD, MEHP University of California, Irvine School of Medicine, Irvine, CA, USA

Michael J. Malinowski, MD, MEHP Division of Vascular Surgery, Medical College of Wisconsin, Milwaukee, WI, USA

Richard G. Milter, PhD, MEd The Johns Hopkins Carey Business School, Baltimore, MD, USA

Sharon K. Park, PharmD, MEHP School of Pharmacy Notre Dame of Maryland University, Baltimore, MD, USA

Juliet M. Ray, EdD, MA Johns Hopkins University School of Education, Baltimore, MD, USA

Bonnie L. Robeson, PhD, MSc, MA The Johns Hopkins Carey Business School, Baltimore, MD, USA

Michael S. Ryan, MD, MEHP Department of Pediatrics, University of Virginia School of Medicine, Charlottesville, VA, USA

Pediatric Hospital Medicine, University of Virginia School of Medicine, Charlottesville, VA, USA

Sean Tackett, MD, MPH Johns Hopkins University School of Medicine, Baltimore, MD, USA

Patricia A. Thomas, MD Department of Medicine, Johns Hopkins University School of Medicine, Baltimore, MD, USA

Serkan Toy, PhD, MEd Departments of Basic Science Education & Health Systems and Implementation Science, Virginia Tech Carilion School of Medicine, Roanoke, VA, USA

Toni Ungaretti, PhD, MSc Masters of Education in the Health Professions (MEHP), Johns Hopkins University School of Education, Baltimore, MD, USA

Kathleen M. White, PhD, MS, RN Johns Hopkins University School of Nursing, Johns Hopkins University School of Education, Baltimore, MD, USA

Julie Youm, PhD, MS, MA University of California, Irvine, School of Medicine, Irvine, CA, USA

Part I
Setting the Stage

Chapter 1
Introduction to Educational Scholarship

April S. Fitzgerald, Gundula Bosch, and Toni Ungaretti

1.1 Introduction

As members of academic medical institutions, many of us have been expected to teach. For health professionals, it can be challenging to balance the need to engage in a primary area of practice while also teaching and providing service to the institution and community. In the past, teaching was viewed by institutions as a necessary but insufficient academic requirement for advancement. This led to teaching being viewed by many as an underappreciated task that was best minimized or avoided in favor of more promotable efforts.

A landmark challenge to this paradigm came in 1990 with the publication of Ernest Boyer's book, "Scholarship Reconsidered: Priorities of the Professoriate."

Boyer's book provided a historical perspective on higher education. He juxtaposed the historical with data detailing the current state of higher education in the late twentieth century.

> Today, when we speak of being "scholarly," it usually means having academic rank in a college or university and being engaged in research and publication. But scholarship in

A. S. Fitzgerald (✉)
Division of General Internal Medicine, Department of Medicine, Johns Hopkins University School of Medicine, Baltimore, MD, USA
e-mail: afitzg10@jhmi.edu

G. Bosch
R3 Center for Innovation in Science Education, Department of Molecular Microbiology and Immunology, Johns Hopkins Bloomberg School of Public Health, Baltimore, MD, USA
e-mail: gbosch2@jhu.edu

T. Ungaretti
Masters of Education in the Health Professions (MEHP), Johns Hopkins University School of Education, Baltimore, MD, USA
e-mail: toni@jhu.edu

© The Author(s), under exclusive license to Springer Nature Switzerland AG 2023
A. S. Fitzgerald, G. Bosch (eds.), *Education Scholarship in Healthcare*, https://doi.org/10.1007/978-3-031-38534-6_1

Table 1.1 Priorities of the professoriate

Boyer's four forms of scholarship
The scholarship of discovery (research)
The scholarship of integration (synthesis)
The scholarship of application (practice)
The scholarship of teaching (education)

earlier times referred to a variety of creative work carried on in a variety of places, and its integrity was measured by the ability to think, communicate, and learn—Ernest Boyer ([1], p 15).

Boyer included teaching as one of the four forms of scholarship: discovery, integration, application, and teaching. He encouraged institutions to reconsider their perspectives of teaching but noted that it is the faculty who bear the responsibility for giving scholarship a more vital meaning. His vision was one where education scholars work collaboratively and creatively. Since its publication, others have continued to build upon Boyer's foundation to clarify and define scholarship as it relates to teaching.

In recent years, both undergraduate and graduate medical education accrediting bodies have recognized and included teaching outcomes in their standards. Beyond *"what are we teaching,"* the accreditors want to see *"what are they learning."* With this shift, the role of health professions teacher has gained more attention, and institutions have begun to recognize the contributions of educational scholarship to the medical professions and to the promotions process (Table 1.1).

1.2 What Is Educational Scholarship

The term education scholarship itself can be confusing. To be *scholarly* indicates that an inquiry is made in a traditional academic way, through the development and testing of a hypothesis. However, the term *scholarship* refers to the dissemination of a scholarly work. When referring to educational scholarship, we are referring to all four forms of Boyer's scholarship in education—discovery (research), integration (synthesis), application (practice), and teaching.

Examples—Have you ever wondered
- If a new instructional strategy might yield better outcomes than a previous one?
- How patient satisfaction will change with the introduction of a new policy?
- How your trainees' self-ratings differ from their demonstrated knowledge?

These are examples of scholarly questions, and there are countless other options and opportunities for educational scholarship investigations. There are several steps once a health scholar decides upon an educational question [2]. First, you need to plan an investigation, then produce the information (data), scrutinize and interpret the findings (and thereby determine whether the results are significant), and, lastly, share these findings with others.

Each step above has multiple smaller steps embedded within. In the final step of sharing your findings with others, dissemination, you typically make suggestions for the next steps, the work is peer-reviewed and made public, and it contributes to the scholarly conversation focused on the creation of new knowledge and its application. This process is critical to a scholarly activity being transformed into educational scholarship. Note that without this last step of sharing significant findings with others—usually a professional audience—this sequence is only considered a scholar*ly* activity, not actual scholar*ship* (Fig. 1.1).

The educational scholarship book can assist you with defining your scholarly interests, choosing a topic and question, and planning your project agenda.

The lifework of an academic health institution includes faculty engagement in what is often characterized as a three-legged stool of the academic mission. It includes one leg for research, one for clinical practice, and one for teaching (Fig. 1.2). While the path to career advancement is usually clearly defined for research activities and clinical practice, the value assigned to teaching varies based on how individual institutions shape their role and reward systems. With the three legs having uneven weight at the institutional level, faculty experience a state of imbalance among the three major missions.

Health professionals are formally supervised in clinical practice before being allowed to provide clinical care independently, and they are taught research methods and mentored before being expected (or allowed) to perform research independently, yet they are often expected to be an educator without the same formal support structure to ensure success in practice and as a scholar.

Understandably, faculty who are given the task of teaching initially approach their assignment as a technical task. As they add teaching or curriculum development to their many competing demands, often without guidance on how to incorporate this work to advance their career, teaching often becomes a time-consuming milestone. Even faculty who enjoy teaching are often discouraged if they have not been given insight into how teaching can enhance their careers.

We want to reconfigure this teaching paradigm for you. Instead of teaching impeding your academic career journey, teaching can be career enhancing.

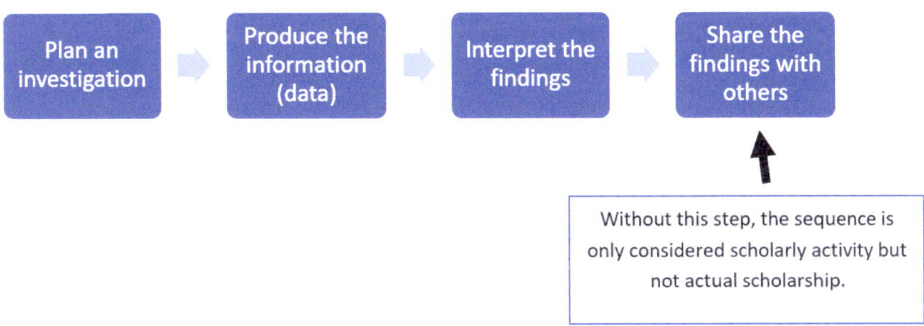

Fig. 1.1 Steps in a scholarship project

Fig. 1.2 Academic medical centers' competing priorities

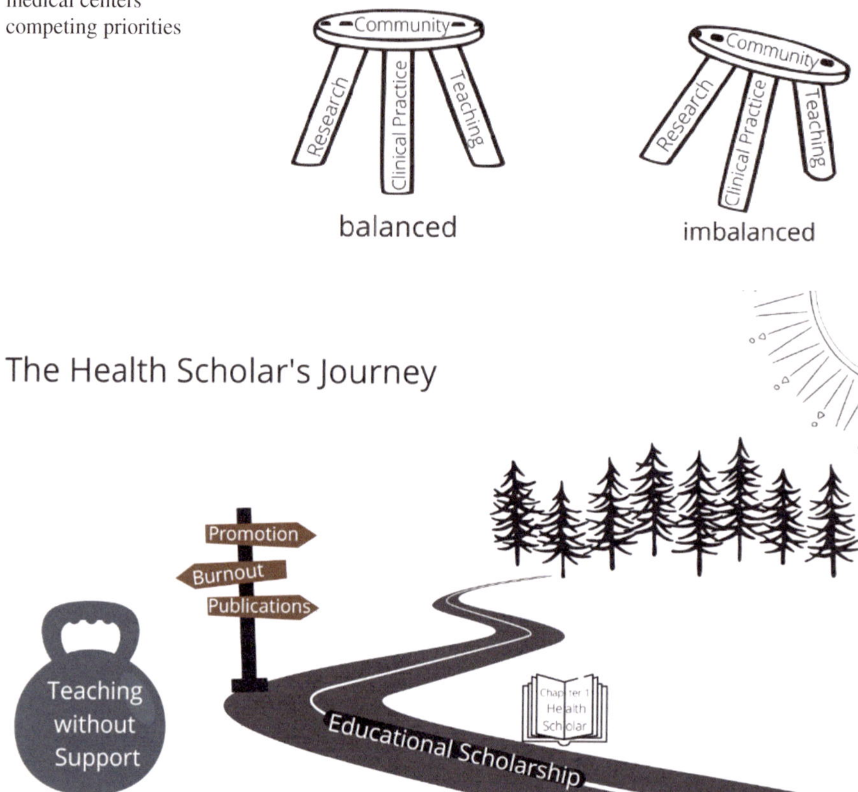

Fig. 1.3 The health scholar's journey

Education scholarship can help you see the benefits of your dedicated efforts, so you can enjoy the journey and avoid derailment or burnout (Fig. 1.3).

1.3 The Benefits of Educational Scholarship

There are many benefits to education scholarship. Below are just a few.

1.3.1 Benefits of Educational Scholarship to the Individual

Academic promotion—It is sometimes thought that faculty who teach are sacrificing time they could be spending elsewhere on a more promotable career advancement opportunity. By learning to reframe teaching as scholarship, faculty earn credit for their work in recognizable academic currency, e.g., scholarship that is recognized within their profession. Disseminated findings on teaching and learning will help faculty gain credibility within their profession, enhance their curriculum vitae with published papers and presentations, and help enhance their reputation. These are all factors used on academic promotion boards.

Being part of an intellectual academic community—This benefit should not be underestimated. It is helpful in academia to find a community of colleagues with whom you have a common purpose and can share ideas. Through communities and collaborations of educational scholars, you will be able to engage in discourse and build on your success and the success of others, while doing work that is impactful and meaningful.

Personal growth—There is personal satisfaction in creating new knowledge and ideas, shaping the future of health care, and joining colleagues who research to advance teaching and education. A record of scholarship in education brings recognition from colleagues and results in additional opportunities to engage with the broader professional community in the research agenda on effective teaching.

1.3.2   Benefits to the Institution

Evidence of continuous quality improvement—A scholarly approach to education keeps in mind the learning outcomes and gathers evidence of their being achieved and approaches to improvement. Teaching is conducted based on the evidence of effective practice and with an orientation toward improvement Published papers bring prestige to the institution. Having published papers speak to the quality of the teaching in individual courses is helpful when it is time for the institution to have its accrediting agency cycle review.

Impact on the learning community—In the end, it is the community that the educator serves that will ultimately benefit from the educational scholarship. The dissemination of the information to a wide audience benefits those you are serving.

1.3.3   Benefits to the Profession

For the profession, educational scholarship creates new knowledge and ideas, advances education for trainees and professionals, and provides insight into questions about our institutions and ourselves that shape the future of health care.

Creating new knowledge and ideas—Education scholarship is the mechanism for the creation of new ideas and new knowledge that keeps progress in motion and stagnation at bay. It is the curious mind and academic process that ensure that we keep moving the field forward.

Advances education for trainees and faculty development—The evidence-based improvement of the educational process is essential to ensure the effective preparation and continuous training of health professionals.

Provides insight into questions about our institutions and ourselves that shape the future of health care—The future of health care relies on an expanded view of teaching and an ability to understand ourselves and our institutions to better prepare the next generation of leaders.

1.4　Defining Educational Scholarship

Different types of educational activities can be philosophically approached as scholarship. The key is to be intentional about creating research questions to pursue in the process of education.

What defines educational scholarship has been examined in the literature. Five broad categories have emerged [3]:

- Teaching
- Learner assessment
- Curriculum development
- Mentoring and advising
- Educational leadership and administration

Questions to ask are: What is the need that is being addressed? What is the gap between the current approach and the ideal approach? What might address that gap? How will the impact of that change be measured? How will the results inform future practice? (Table 1.2).

Table 1.2 Five categories of educator contributions from AAMC GEA [3]

Teaching	Any activity that fosters learning, including direct teaching and the creation of associated instructional materials
Learner assessment	All activities associated with measuring learners' knowledge, skills, and attitudes related to one or more of the following activities: development, implementation, analysis, or synthesis and presentation
Curriculum development	A longitudinal set that is more than one teaching session or presentation of designed educational activities that includes evaluation, which may occur at any training level
Mentoring and advising	Mentoring: a sustained, committed relationship from which both parties obtain reciprocal benefits. Advising: a more limited relationship than mentoring that usually occurs over a limited period, with the advisor serving as a guide
Educational leadership and administration	Achieving results through others, transforming organizations through the vigorous pursuit of excellence with their work's value demonstrated through ongoing evaluation, dissemination of results, and maximization of resources

Simpson, D., & Anderson, M. B. (2006). Educational Scholarship: How do we define and acknowledge it? *Medical Education. Feb*

1.5 How This Book Is Organized

The first section of the book, Chaps. 1–2, introduces the health scholar to the rationale for scholarship. Chap. 2 will introduce you to Glassick's criteria for scholarship and describe some common types of scholarship in health educational practice. You will learn the notion of a scholarship niche as an individual health educator's specific area of scholarly interest. We will ask you to think about your own educational research niche.

The second section of the book, Chaps. 3–5, is methods based. It starts with the concept of *gap in the literature* and the literature review. You will find some strategies such as the annotated bibliography that can help with tackling the vast amount of information that you might find in your area of interest. Then you will explore why research methods matter and what are the conceptual building blocks of research. Each reader should think about their own educational research interest as they read through the sections. You can consider how to answer your research question using approaches such as qualitative, qualitative, and mixed-methods research.

The third section of the book, Chaps. 6–8, looks at paradigms, outcomes, and ethics. Starting with evaluation paradigms that might be used for thinking about a medical scholarship question—Bloom's taxonomy, Kirkpatrick's model of evaluation, Miller's pyramid, and the validity evidence model—the section moves into exploring the variables being addressed in the question. Looking at the variables and the evaluation paradigms, the outcomes chapter discusses the impact of educational research and the alignment of the research question, methodology, and outcomes. Then, we are introduced to the importance of ethics in research and how the institutional review board (IRB) for institutions safeguards the human subject research process. This is a fascinating part of educational scholarship that the health scholar will appreciate.

The fourth section of the book, Chaps. 9–13, is the dissemination section of the book. It gets to the heart of where and how you disseminate your work by first exploring what portion of educational work might be appropriate for dissemination and how to position educational work for publication. The section then discusses the types of abstracts that can be written for an educational scholarship project and the details of how to write an abstract. Next is a focus on an introduction to the medical research poster, an important vehicle for sharing scholarly work with the medical community, followed by the mechanics of writing a manuscript that will be submitted for publication. The section wraps up with peer review with the purpose of the peer-review process discussed in the context of dissemination of educational scholarship. The last chapter also provides guidelines for serving in the role of reviewer.

The fifth section of the book, Chaps. 14–17, looks at the work behind the scenes. It will help you with the important questions of how you do the work that will yield the results you will be disseminating. The section starts by exploring the myriad of logistics necessary to consider when contemplating an educational scholarship project. Project planning includes such items as personnel, time, facilities, equipment, instruments, expenses, support, and buy-in from stakeholders. The section then moves on to explore which aspects of your work will result in costs and how to find support. It will then explore what it means to have a "culture of mentorship" in the professional environment and what makes an effective mentor for educational and/or scholarly work. The chapter will also explore *traditional* mentors, *functional* mentors, and *facilitators* and how they support the health scholar in addressing barriers to scholarly project completion. The last chapter in the section will discuss some basic principles of leadership needed in any environment.

The final section of the book, Chap. 18, brings additional depth to topics for the interested reader.

1.6 Conclusion

We will guide you to use what you are already doing in your professional practice so it can be transformed into a scholarly project with a bit of a structured approach. Becoming a scholar is less difficult than you may think, and one does not need to be a formal classroom teacher or academic researcher to produce education scholarship. We welcome you. This book has been written in a spirit of authenticity and collaboration hoping to create an environment where you, the reader, will feel comfortable. We appreciate the faith you have placed in us as guides on this journey, and we hope to fulfill your needs. We are delighted to be on this journey with you.

1.7 Questions

Discussion
1. What is educational scholarship, and what elements are critical to it?

Activities
1. Based on the chapter information and your interests, list initial ideas for broad topics of educational scholarship that interest you.

    (a) Why are you interested in that topic?
    (b) How might this topic impact your career?

2. What are some of the work demands that present challenges to your scholarship production?

    (a) What strategies and approaches might help you effectively address these challenges or turn them into avenues for scholarship?

References

1. Boyer EL. Scholarship reconsidered: priorities of the professoriate. Princeton: Princeton University Press; 1990.
2. Lambert M. A beginner's guide to doing your education research project. Thousand Oaks: Sage; 2012.
3. Simpson D, Anderson MB. Educational scholarship: how do we define and acknowledge it? Washington, DC: AAMC; 2006. https://www.aamc.org/professional-development/affinity-groups/gfa/faculty-vitac/definingeducational-scholarship

Chapter 2
Introduction to Education Research

Sharon K. Park, Khanh-Van Le-Bucklin, and Julie Youm

2.1 Introduction

The probing mind of the researcher is an incalculably vital asset to the academy and the world. Scholarly investigation, in all the disciplines, is at the very heart of academic life, and the pursuit of knowledge must be assiduously cultivated and defended. The intellectual excitement fueled by this quest enlivens faculty and invigorates higher learning institutions, and in our complicated, vulnerable world, the discovery of new knowledge is absolutely crucial—Ernest Boyer [1].

Research is defined by the Oxford English Dictionary as "the systematic investigation into and study of materials and sources in order to establish facts and reach new conclusions." Inv the health sciences, research is routinely conducted across the basic, clinical, and translational sciences with established and understood levels of rigor and methodological approaches that are universally recognized as systematic investigations. However, research in the field of health professions education, and education in general, is far more contested, largely due to the conflicting perspectives around education, the paradigms used to study it, and the diversity of disciplines encompassed [2]. Despite this, the "discovery of new knowledge is absolutely crucial" as stated by Ernest Boyer, a past President at the Carnegie Foundation for the Advancement of Teaching. Education research must prevail so that advances and innovation for our learners can be informed by true evidence-based knowledge and practices.

S. K. Park (✉)
School of Pharmacy, Notre Dame of Maryland University, Baltimore, MD, USA
e-mail: spark@ndm.edu

K.-V. Le-Bucklin · J. Youm
University of California, Irvine School of Medicine, Irvine, CA, USA
e-mail: klebuckl@uci.edu; jyoum@uci.edu

A. S. Fitzgerald, G. Bosch (eds.), *Education Scholarship in Healthcare*, https://doi.org/10.1007/978-3-031-38534-6_2

13

This chapter aims to introduce the basics of education research to promote systematic investigations in the field. The importance and role of research for health professions education will be discussed from the perspective of supporting both the learner and the educator. Key definitions and the cycle of scholarship will be described using Glassick's criteria.

2.2 The Benefits of Education Research

Educators rely on the discovery of new knowledge about teaching practices and frameworks to improve and evolve education for trainees. Decisions around curricular change require thoughtful consideration about how to integrate this new knowledge, as they can have significant impacts on learner performance, achievement of program objectives, and compliance with accreditation standards. In health professions education, the ultimate goal of graduating competent healthcare providers carries the additional stipulation that the quality of an educational program will have a direct influence on patient outcomes. In this way, research focused on health professions education benefits and influences learners first and foremost, and subsequently, patients as beneficiaries of successful learner achievement.

Education research can also provide benefits to the educator as well as to the institution. Educators in higher education apply new knowledge gained from research in the field to improve their own teaching and evaluations. Educators benefit from conducting education research that yields publications and scholarship, which can be used to gain promotions and tenure, recognition in their field, and a place in the community of health professions scholars [3]. Additionally, institutions use education research to establish support for the allocation of resources to instructional activities or to obtain funding for new initiatives and technologies [3]. When determining resource allocation, faculty development for education research is vital to the success of not only the faculty themselves but also the learners and the profession at large. Because a majority of health professions faculty are clinicians, it is important and necessary to recognize the nuances and unique aspects of education research when compared with clinical or basic science research.

2.3 Definitions in Education Research

Education research is a scientific process that involves methodologies that promote a systematic and objective outcome. The process starts with the articulation of a phenomenon of interest or a problem to be solved. The problem is then formulated into a research question that informs the goals and objectives of a study.

In the development of the research question, it must be determined if the question is "researchable": if it is important and will contribute to what is already known in the field. Constructing a conceptual framework is a critical step in helping to situate and explicitly connect the research question to literature in the field [4]. "A conceptual framework is the justification for why a given study should be conducted. The conceptual framework (1) describes the state of known knowledge, usually through a literature review; (2) identifies gaps in our understanding of a phenomenon or problem; and (3) outlines the methodological underpinnings of the research project" [5]. Thus, a conceptual framework defines both the reason (why answering the research question matters) and the rigor (why the research methodology is appropriate), for the research at hand [6].

2.3.1 Methodologies

The construction of a conceptual framework plays an important role in selecting an appropriate research methodology for a study. An education research methodology represents how the research is designed and conducted to meet the study objectives with valid and reliable results. A broad view of education research methodology distinguishes three primary types:

- Quantitative research
- Qualitative research
- Mixed-methods research

2.3.2 Research Approaches

"Research approaches articulate the plans and decisions that outline the process from study formation to methodologies involved in data collection, analysis, and interpretation" [7]. While research approaches are often characterized by methodologies that are based on the type of data involved, there exist further principles that influence the decisions a researcher makes in determining the scope and direction of a scientific study (as presented in [7]):

- Philosophical assumptions (research paradigm or philosophies of science)
- Research designs (processes of inquiry)
- Research methods (data collection, analysis, and interpretation)

Later chapters will provide further details on the philosophies of science, research designs, and research methodologies. For those initiating education research, awareness of the essential components of research approaches and understanding their relationship in establishing the standards of rigor for a scientific study will help advance the field of health professions education through a lens towards quality contributions.

2.4 Scholarship Niche

An important consideration that should be made when embarking on a career conducting education research is finding a scholarship niche, "a specialized corner of your field—where you could conduct research for the next 10 years or so to make the greatest impact" [8]. In other words, how do you want to distinguish yourself from the rest of the field? You may find that your scholarship niche for education research is distinct from your established clinical, basic science, and/or translational scholarship niches.

If applying for a grant and funding opportunities, your credentials, publications, and presentations will help to establish your research qualifications. By conducting a self-assessment of your scholarship portfolio and taking on the perspective of a future peer reviewer, you will be able to see where your expertise stands out. Similarly, ask trusted colleagues and mentors to provide a thoughtful and critical assessment of your scholarship as well.

Researchers often stay in the field where they are working and/or in one that is very closely related. However, once you have gained experience conducting research, successful past performance can signal potential for future success if pursuing new areas of research is desired.

In finding the scholarship niche that is right for you, reflect on the following (adapted from [9]):

- Identify the most promising research needs and opportunities in the field.
- Evaluate the competitive landscape; know who is doing what and which research approaches they employ.
- Assess whether you have the knowledge base and skills to perform cutting-edge research that will make an impact.

When shifting from a general area of research to a more specialized one, it is important to learn as much about the broader field as possible. Networking is one way to achieve this goal. Seek out those in your local institution with a demonstrated depth of experience. Seek out those outside your institution who present at scientific meetings, specialty-specific conferences, and other educational forums. Review the literature for hot topics and knowledge gaps that can provide opportunities for your contribution and impact in the field. Finally, once you have identified a scholarship niche to pursue, assess again your knowledge and skills to be successful in moving the field forward.

2.5 Glassick's Criteria for Education Scholarship

In response to Ernest Boyer's seminal report *"Scholarship Reconsidered: Priorities of the Professoriate"* (see Chap. 1), Glassick et al. [10] conducted research about the criteria and decision processes for grants and publications. The remarkable finding from this study was the level to which responses shared overarching themes. The analysis of these themes resulted in the derivation of six standards, known as Glassick's criteria, that can be used to assess all forms of scholarship.

The standards defined in Glassick's criteria provide a tangible measure by which educators can assess the quality and structure of their education research. While these standards are often discussed in the context of evaluating the scholarship of discovery, such as in traditional research, it is important to keep in mind that these six standards can be applied across all four of Boyer's forms of scholarship. Case examples of the application of these criteria can be found in the Appendix section.

2.5.1 Standard 1: Clear Goals

- Does the scholar state the basic purpose of his or her work clearly?
- Does the scholar define objectives that are realistic and achievable?
- Does the scholar identify important questions in the field?

Setting clear goals is an important step in conducting education research that can only happen after one has a sufficient understanding of a problem. Often, this first step can take the longest time to develop compared with the rest of the criteria. Goals are often achieved through an iterative effort to understand what is known and what is unknown, as well as understanding the significance of investigating the problem to the field [11]. Without this effort, hastily decided research goals and objectives can lead to expending additional time and resources at a cost to the research team, institution, and learners. The mismatch between the objectives and all other parts of the research may lead to a midway modification, a restart, or a waste of precious resources already spent.

When research is set to begin, these questions should be answered with relative confidence
- Who will be the beneficiaries of this research?
- What is the current gap in knowledge in the literature about this topic?
- What is the ultimate goal of this research or what can it offer to learners, instructors, or institutions?
- How long would this research take from the beginning (idea conceptualization) to the outcomes manifested by learners?
- When would be an optimal time to begin the research?

Answering these questions honestly and thoughtfully will help elucidate concerns about the rigor and relevance of the research. When setting clear goals, researchers should strive for clarity in their hypotheses and achievable, measurable objectives in their work [12].

2.5.2 Standard 2: Adequate Preparation

- Does the scholar show an understanding of existing scholarship in the field?
- Does the scholar bring the necessary skills to his or her work?
- Does the scholar bring together the resources necessary to move the project forward?

Education research should be based on current and existing scholarship with research questions and hypotheses grounded in known conceptual and theoretical frameworks. This is achieved by having adequate preparation for research efforts before they begin. Adequate preparation can include thorough literature reviews and consultation with content and methodological experts [12]. Recognizing the limitations of available resources (e.g., time, people, technology) is critical to constructing objectives that can be accomplished within those limits.

Once the research objectives are determined, the following questions should be addressed before moving forward
- What are some of the key background literature and current knowledge on this topic?
- If there is a lot of information in the literature, how selective should the focus be and how much time should be dedicated to this part given the focus?
- Is there any additional training necessary to begin or strengthen any part of this research (e.g., updating certification for human research training)?
- What types of support or resources are available to successfully meet the research goals? Would having a statistician be helpful or necessary?
- Who should be consulted and be aware of my research endeavors in my institution?
- Who are my target learners (e.g., subjects) for this research, and do I have access to them?
- Would approval from the institutional review board be required for this research? If so, how long does it typically take to receive one?
- Who should I select as a mentor or someone as a guiding "second set of eyes and ears" to ensure its success?
- What are ethical and procedural policies within the institution that should be followed?

2.5.3 Standard 3: Appropriate Methods

- Does the scholar use methods appropriate to the goals?
- Does the scholar apply effectively the methods selected?
- Does the scholar modify procedures in response to changing circumstances?

The methods implemented for an educational research study should align with its set goals and objectives. This means ensuring that a proposed study design can answer the research question and that the statistical analyses are appropriate [12]. When designing a research study and determining its research methods, the following questions should be addressed:

- What are the measurable outcomes of this research?
- Which research design best fits the outcomes?
- How would you measure the outcomes, quantitatively, qualitatively, or both? If both, which part of the measurements requires quantitative or qualitative methods?
- How appropriate are these methods? Is there a more appropriate method that would require a consultation from an expert or a statistician?
- Does the research method capture all aspects of the expected outcomes? Are there gaps in accounting for any confounding variables?
- What are the anticipated limitations or weaknesses of this research that can possibly be amended or strengthened?
- What are the expected outcomes that would warrant consideration before starting?
- How should any potential bias be managed?
- If any biases cannot be eliminated based on the chosen research method, how would the outcomes be affected and anticipated to change?

Research often presents an evaluation or a measurement that is not congruent with the expected outcome. For example, a multiple-choice test of a learner's knowledge-based competencies may not demonstrate the clinical skill competencies achieved as an expected outcome for a procedure-based curricular intervention.

2.5.4 *Standard 4: Significant Result*

- Does the scholar achieve the goals?
- Does the scholar's work add consequentially to the field?
- Does the scholar's work open additional areas for further exploration?

Significance from a research perspective is the degree to which the results of the work met the goals set forth. This could be measured by the magnitude of the results, the statistical significance of any quantitative results, and the implications for the findings in the field [11]. When collecting and analyzing data to determine study outcomes, the following questions should be addressed:

- How best should data be presented (e.g., tables, graphs, confidence intervals)?
- How should these data be interpreted? Did the data adequately explain the research question and hypothesis?
- If qualitative analysis was performed, did the data identify salient themes in the results? If mixed methods were used, were the results triangulated to draw conclusions?

- Were there any unexpected outcomes emerging from the data? Were they relevant to answering the question?
- How do the results of this study help advance the field? How are they not helpful or inadequate to answer other questions?
- What are the strengths of this study that can contribute to other research questions?

2.5.5 Standard 5: Effective Presentation

- Does the scholar use a suitable style and effective organization to present his or her work?
- Does the scholar use appropriate forums for communicating the work to its intended audiences?
- Does the scholar present his or her message with clarity and integrity?

Effective presentation and dissemination of scholarship are vital for advancing any field. Opportunities for effective presentation include lectures, podcasts, academic journals, professional meetings and conferences, and educational repositories. For educational research to be recognized as scholarship, the work must be public, peer-reviewed, and disseminated in a form that allows others to build on it [13].

When preparing for a presentation either in written or in verbal formats, the following questions should be considered
- Who is the target audience?
- What resources does the presentation require? If presenting at a meeting, does it require a pre-meeting submission and need to meet the criteria for continuing education?
- What is the requirement for length of presentation in time (minutes, hours) or pages (word count)?
- Are figures and tables necessary to convey the results effectively and efficiently? If so, what are the limits in the number and size?
- Given the data types and analyses, what is the most appropriate method of presenting them (e.g., quantitative vs. qualitative, mean vs. median vs. mode, standard deviation vs. range)?
- Which type of graphical methods should be used (e.g., pie chart, scatterplot)?
- How should a summary or conclusion be presented or written to convey the main points?

2.5.6 Standard 6: Reflective Critique

- Does the scholar critically evaluate his or her own work?

- Does the scholar bring an appropriate breadth of evidence to his or her critique?
- Does the scholar use evaluation to improve the quality of future work?

The last step in the education research process is to engage in a critical reflection of the results and implications in light of the literature and any limitations to guide the direction of future work [11]. After completing research and publishing its results, it may seem prudent to consider moving promptly to new or other pending projects. However, it is critical to reexamine the completed research to objectively evaluate the process and results to improve future endeavors, large or small.

When critiquing the study, the following questions should be considered
- What are the implications of this study's result to the overall discipline, knowledge, or field of research?
- What are the limitations of this study that could have contributed to not accomplishing the research goal?
- How could the study have been designed, executed, or implemented to better address the method?
- What possibilities exist to interpret the results in unintended or negative implications?
- Should the research question be considered answered or still open to discussion and further exploration?
- What is the quality of the study? How was this quality determined?
- How could this quality level be improved for an increased external validity (e.g., sample size, statistical rigor)?

Addressing these questions will not only help educators improve on their research skills and strategies for the future, but also help them realize that there is always further growth and development in education research no matter the rigor or resources put into the current study. This reflection propels the researcher to continue to ask further questions and seek appropriate methods to answer them down the road.

2.6 Conclusion

This chapter introduced the basics of education research to promote systematic investigations in the field. Key definitions and the cycle of scholarship were presented as well as an overview of the six Glassick's criteria. Case examples were presented to better describe how Glassick's criteria can be applied in real-life research and scholarship process. Education research should be an important component of a scholarly instructor; therefore, instructors are encouraged to apply Glassick's criteria to assess their ongoing or future research endeavors so that their efforts are thoroughly executed and meaningfully translated to sharable and impactful scholarship.

2.7 Questions

Discussion Questions

1. What big-picture label would encompass your area of interest?
   Example: policy, organizational structure, evaluation, instructional strategies, and learner characteristics
2. Does your area of interest need narrowing down to truly be a niche? If yes, how could you do that?

Activities

1. In your area of educational interest, list an example of each of the following:

   (a) A performance measure
   (b) A program evaluation
   (c) An evidence-based policy or practice

2. Think about a pressing question in your work that interests you:

   (a) What information would help you answer the question?
   (b) How would you use that information?

References

1. Boyer EL. Scholarship reconsidered: priorities of the professoriate. Princeton: Carnegie Foundation for the Advancement of Teaching; 1990.
2. Munoz-Najar Galvez S, Heiberger R, McFarland D. Paradigm wars revisited: a cartography of graduate research in the field of education (1980–2010). Am Educ Res J. 2020;57(2):612–52.
3. Ringsted C, Hodges B, Scherpbier A. 'The research compass': an introduction to research in medical education: AMEE Guide no. 56. Med Teach. 2011;33(9):695–709.
4. Bordage G. Conceptual frameworks to illuminate and magnify. Med Educ. 2009;43(4):312–9.
5. Varpio L, Paradis E, Uijtdehaage S, Young M. The distinctions between theory, theoretical framework, and conceptual framework. Acad Med. 2020;95(7):989–94.
6. Ravitch SM, Riggins M. Reason & Rigor: how conceptual frameworks guide research. Thousand Oaks: Sage Publications; 2017.
7. Park YS, Zaidi Z, O'Brien BC. RIME foreword: what constitutes science in educational research? Applying rigor in our research approaches. Acad Med. 2020;95(11S):S1–5.
8. National Institute of Allergy and Infectious Diseases. Writing a winning application—You're your niche. 2020a. https://www.niaid.nih.gov/grants-contracts/find-your-niche. Accessed 23 Jan 2022.
9. National Institute of Allergy and Infectious Diseases. Writing a winning application—conduct a self-assessment. 2020b. https://www.niaid.nih.gov/grants-contracts/winning-app-self-assessment. Accessed 23 Jan 2022.
10. Glassick CE, Huber MT, Maeroff GI. Scholarship assessed: evaluation of the professoriate. San Francisco: Jossey Bass; 1997.
11. Simpson D, Meurer L, Braza D. Meeting the scholarly project requirement-application of scholarship criteria beyond research. J Grad Med Educ. 2012;4(1):111–2. https://doi.org/10.4300/JGME-D-11-00310.1.

12. Fincher RME, Simpson DE, Mennin SP, Rosenfeld GC, Rothman A, McGrew MC et al. The council of academic societies task force on scholarship. Scholarship in teaching: an imperative for the 21st century. Academic Medicine. 2000;75(9):887–94.
13. Hutchings P, Shulman LS. The scholarship of teaching new elaborations and developments. Change. 1999;11–5.

Part II
Laying the Foundation

Chapter 3
Reviewing the Literature

Ahmed Ibrahim

3.1 Introduction

An important premise of this chapter is that a health scholar must first grasp what exists in the literature before producing scholarship. Boote and Beile ([1], p 3) describe this premise: "A substantive, thorough, sophisticated literature review is a precondition for doing substantive, thorough, sophisticated research." A thorough review of the literature has importance and value because it is the foundation of your future work. Like the concrete and steel foundation that supports the physical structure of a building, the foundation for a scholarship project is layered knowledge that is cumulative and supportive.

During the review, you might find enlightened ideas that you agree with, or you might find some specific ideas, stances, or conclusions that you do not agree with. Either way, it is important to know the existence of these layers before attempting to build upon them. Prior works can add knowledge by highlighting limitations of procedure or thought. You might also find gaps or criticisms of a prior research frontier. Highly scrutinized peer-reviewed prior work will help you think through how to move forward.

In their eagerness for scholarship, some new scholars have asked research questions, collected/analyzed data, and written manuscripts without having a good understanding of the existing literature. The result is unhappy. Without understanding what came before, an investigation may result in work yielding a suboptimal contribution or no meaningful impact. The work is rejected or unappreciated because it failed to reveal new insights or acknowledge prior work. The literature review necessitates holding a high priority as a precondition for research and a foundation for producing scholarship.

A. Ibrahim (✉)
Johns Hopkins University School of Education, Baltimore, MD, USA
e-mail: aibrahim@jhu.edu

© The Author(s), under exclusive license to Springer Nature Switzerland AG 2023

A. S. Fitzgerald, G. Bosch (eds.), *Education Scholarship in Healthcare*, https://doi.org/10.1007/978-3-031-38534-6_3

Other scholars submit outstanding work but fail to explicitly identify their conceptual framework. The conceptual framework allows the health scholar to identify the importance of the work. Without an explicitly stated framework, attempts at publication can similarly yield unhappy results. A thorough review of the literature is necessary to clarify theory and frameworks as part of early project development [2].

In this chapter, I hope to help you recognize the high value of performing a substantive, thorough, sophisticated literature review so you can avoid such pitfalls. We will look at the literature review's importance for the engagement and production of scholarship as well as its benefits for self-development and your career. By recognizing the crucial role that a literature review plays as a precondition for conducting and producing meaningful investigations, health scholars and their community can emphasize the value of contributing significant scholarship that advances knowledge with impact.

3.2 The Benefits of Reviewing the Literature

Literature reviews have been found to increase publications, which in turn leads to increased opportunities and improved competitiveness for grants, awards, and employment among early-career researchers [3]. The health scholar who does a thorough review of the literature quickly becomes a comparative expert in the field. In addition to the self-satisfaction of learning about a subject of interest, the increase in knowledge base can raise the profile of the health scholar in the community to which they belong. This alone can lead to multiple opportunities for collaboration or engagement in professional activities in which expertise is sought.

The impact of understanding the literature and conducting a review is not limited to health scholars who seek publication. A thirst for knowledge and the ability to conduct a thorough literature review should be a comfortable competency of students, teachers, administrators, and leaders. Boote and Beile [1] described knowing the literature as a "responsibility" that, no matter which role the health scholar has, is something required from us. As professionals in our fields of expertise or as students on a path to develop such expertise, to engage in meaningful dialogues, to join conversations with intelligence and wit, or to contribute to knowledge and have an impact, it is necessary to understand the literature in a deep sophisticated manner.

The literature review can be developed in several ways and presented in different formats.

- As in *Introduction*: A common format for the literature review is the Introduction section of a manuscript. The review serves the purpose of introducing the reader to the subject area and highlighting the need for the manuscript's topic by orienting the reader to a literature gap or a specific problem. In this case, the literature review tends to be brief and succinct yet written in a way that elegantly summarizes the existing work.

- As a *Standalone Paper*: Another format for the literature review is as a complete paper dedicated solely to presenting the body of literature in a specific area of study. In this case, the literature review tends to be expansive and elaborate. It usually presents all the details of conducting the review. Since there are limitations on the number of words or pages in a publication, the steps that were followed in conducting the review are sometimes included in separate appendices or online supplementary materials.

3.3 Theory and Frameworks

Health scholars are often asked about the theory and frameworks upon which their scholarship is anchored, and the decisions regarding dissemination might be determined by their answers. These terms—theory, framework, conceptual framework, and theoretical framework—can be confusing and are sometimes used interchangeably.

As part of a large collection exploring the philosophy of science, Varpio [4] helped to address some of the confusion that exists in the health professions education (HPE) literature surrounding these terms with the following definitions [4]:

- *Theory*—an abstract description of relationships between concepts that helps in understanding the world (Table 3.1).
- *Theoretical framework*—a logically developed and connected set of concepts and premises developed from one or more theories that a health scholar uses to support a project.
- *Conceptual framework*—the justification for why a study/project was conducted. It includes (1) current state of knowledge, (2) gap in understanding, and (3) method of the project (Table 3.2).

Table 3.1 Types of theories

Theory type	What it is	Examples
Descriptive	Describes how things really are rather than how they should be	Naming, characterizing
Explanatory	Make sense of complex situations	Clarifying relationships
Emancipatory	Identifies a central moral purpose for the production of knowledge	Articulating the oppression of people
Disruptive	Science copes and thrives on unstable ground	Extending or refuting the existing knowledge
Predictive	Generating testable predictions	Predicting an outcome based on an input

Adapted from Varpio, L., Paradis, E., Uijtdehaage, S., & Young, M. (2020). The distinctions between theory, theoretical framework, and conceptual framework. *Academic Medicine*, 95(7), 989-994

Table 3.2 Common conceptual frameworks in HPE

Conceptual framework	Attributed to	Example application
Deliberate practice	Ericsson	Simulation-based curriculum Skill acquisition over time
Automaticity and skill expertise	Fitts and Posner	Procedural skill acquisition
Cognitive load theory	Sweller, Van Merrienboer, and Paas	Design of handouts and slides
Self-directed learning	Knowles	Individualized learning plans
Social cognitive theory	Bandura	Discussion boards
Self-regulated learning	Zimmerman and Schunk	Self-directed goals
Reflective practice	Schon	Reflective writing
Self-determination	Deci and Ryan	Problem-based learning, small-group learning
Experiential learning cycle	Kolb	Staggered learning sessions
Situated learning-guided participation	Vygotsky	Workshops

Adapted from Zackoff, M. W., Real, F. J., Abramson, E. L., Li, S. T. T., Klein, M. D., & Gusic, M. E. (2019). Enhancing educational scholarship through conceptual frameworks: a challenge and roadmap for medical educators. *Academic Pediatrics*, *19*(2), 135-141

When a conceptual framework is used by many researchers, it can help build the strength of understanding behind the framework itself and make it more apparent how ideas translate to other areas (Table 3.2).

3.4 Broad Goals in Reviewing the Literature

Creswell and Guetterman ([5], p 79) defined a review of the literature as "a written summary of journal articles, books, and other documents that describe the past and current state of information on the topic of your research study."

Consider the review as three concentric circles as shown in Fig. 3.1. The first broad circle sets boundaries to include specific studies that define the context of the review. In the middle circle, the review synthesizes the literature and finds trends in the current scholarship. In the innermost circle, the review identifies problems or gaps that need to be addressed. A successful review should go deep into the innermost circle, identifying problems and gaps that can be accompanied by recommendations for future research.

Fig. 3.1 The broad goals reviewing the literature

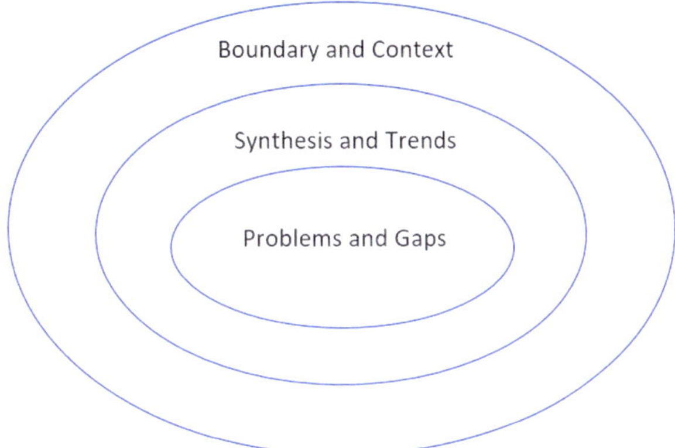

3.4.1 Setting a Boundary and Context

The literature review draws a clear *boundary* around a set of works (studies or publications) that are considered the literature of interest. In such a way, it defines the boundaries and limits for what belongs and what does not belong within the exploration or review of a topic. Of course, this boundary setting is defined by the researcher based on keywords, search strategies, and inclusion/exclusion criteria. These limitations identify the pool of studies that define the literature.

Boote and Beile ([1], p 4) described the review of the literature as "set[ting] the broad context of the study." The word *context* can be vague, but essentially what a literature review does is to clearly identify the set of studies that will be included in a review and those that will not. The studies that are included collectively have certain characteristics that define the scholarly context from different angles such as demographics, research methods, historical, and geographical settings. The studies that are excluded also collectively refer to the external world outside the boundaries of that specific literature review.

The health scholar should be able to describe the theory used in decisions and the relationship between ideas, statements, and concepts. Although the literature review focuses on what is included, it should also situate the review within a broader academic context by explaining links to other areas that are not included in the review. For example, if a literature review focuses on the effects of reading using tablet devices, the world outside that specific literature review could include reading on printed paper. A good literature review should make the link to the outside world of reading on printed paper and describe how it is related to the inside world of reading on tablet devices.

3.4.2 Provides Synthesis and Trends

Another purpose of the literature review is to examine individual studies or papers and group papers based on common themes to get an understanding and a summarization of what has been done, researched, or developed in the past. One important and essential objective of the literature review is to provide a *synthesis*, beyond mere summarization of the collection of sources garnered from the search. This is the collection that we identified as the body of literature that we want to review and represents what lies within the boundary of our review, and again defines the context of our review. The synthesis of the literature should not only summarize the literature but go beyond that and give insights about what can be learned from the summary. A good literature review shows *trends* and patterns in the body of works examined.

In this way, the scholar forms a theoretical framework that explains and supports the planned educational project. The theoretical framework should answer the question, *"How does this theory shape the study?"* [4].

3.4.3 Why is this Research Important?

A health scholar might have a problem in mind and start a review to explore the specific topic in more depth, look for the relationship between variables, or find the effects of an intervention, but the review process itself might reveal insights about unsolved problems that the scholar might not yet have considered. Thus, one of the outcomes or objectives of conducting a literature review is to *identify problems* and deepen the understanding of them. These underlying issues that the scholar identifies can be practical or theoretical in nature and lead to questions and areas of research that need more exploration, the identified *gap*.

From the logically developed need for more exploration, the scholar has identified the conceptual framework of the study, which answers the question, *"Why is this research important?"* [4].

3.5 Types of Gaps: Areas Neglected in the Literature

Research on literature reviews by Sandberg and Alvesson [6] found neglected areas of the existing literature as "the most common mode of constructing research questions." So, why is it important to present and show clearly where it is and how it is something that needed attention and exploration? The astute scholar understands that finding and filling a gap can lead to successful scholarship dissemination and more opportunities for discovery in the future.

Sandberg and Alvesson [6] and Lingard [7] categorize these gaps in the literature into five categories.

1. Overlooked: a gap in the current state of research—This gap is one that has been ignored and not researched in the past. We can think of research that investigates overlooked areas to help us deepen our knowledge in a confined area of research. It is possible to think of this as a gap in the middle of an ongoing research program or line of inquiry.
2. Extension-based: a gap at the forefront—This gap type is for extending and complementing existing literature. The extension-based gap is an area of knowledge that is at the forefront of research. It is not an area that was overlooked or ignored. It is something to complement and add to current research. It is possible to think of this as a gap at the forefront of a research program or line of inquiry.
3. Needing empirical support: a gap in the past—An area with a lack of empirical support is an area in which there are proposed theories and explanatory frameworks or models; however, there is no empirical evidence. Lingard [7] characterized this kind of gap as pervasive and unproven assumptions. It is possible to think of this as a gap in the past, simply because past assumptions were not supported by evidence.
4. Under-researched: An under-researched area is an area that did not receive enough attention and investigation, although some research has already explored some questions in it.
5. Confusion: a lot of research with competing explanations—This gap type is an area where there is a controversy or disagreement among scholars. In many cases, the literature is full of contradictory views and evidence. For example, there are opposite results to the effects of reading on digital devices. Some literature supports that they are better than reading on paper, and some literature shows evidence for the contrary. Some literature also shows no difference. This is an example of a gap in the literature in which there is confusion and controversy (Table 3.3).

Table 3.3 Proposed continuum for research gaps

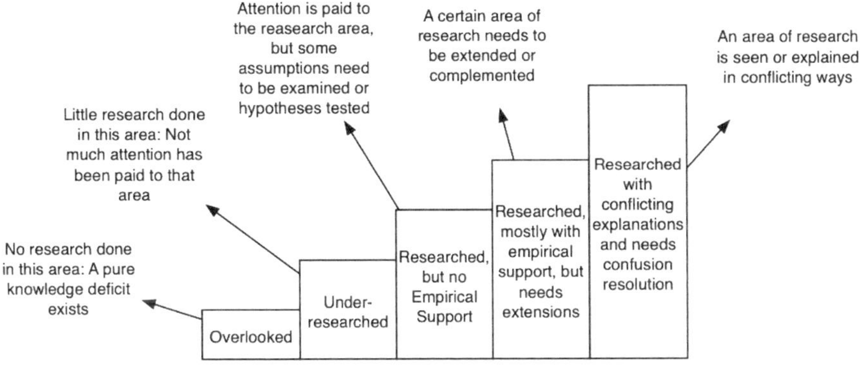

Types of Gaps based on Amount of Research

3.6 The Types of Literature Reviews

We have talked about literature reviews in general terms, but literature reviews come in many shapes and forms. It helps if the health scholar understands the differences so they can select a literature review type that best aligns with their objectives. The nature of the question being asked will be the driving force behind the selection of the type of literature review. This, in turn, will determine the approach, norms, and procedures of the review. Flowing from the type of review decision will be the quantity of resources (time, money, manpower, etc.) that will be needed to accomplish the task.

Paré et al. [8] developed a typology of literature reviews. In their typology, they described four overarching goals for literature reviews—summarization of prior knowledge, data aggregation or integration, explanation building, and critical assessment of extant literature. See Fig. 3.2.

For each overarching goal, there are specific types of literature reviews that fall within it. A health scholar should first decide the goal of the literature review. Using the typology of review, the next step is to choose from the types of literature reviews that fall within that specific goal. For example, if the goal of the review is to summarize a body of literature, then a narrative, descriptive, or scoping review would be appropriate to consider.

3.6.1 Goal: Summarization of Prior Knowledge

- *Narrative Review*: Describes what has been reported in the literature based on a selective sample of publications. This type of review is what is frequently included in the introductions of research articles that try to selectively summarize previous relevant research.

Overarching Goal of Literature Review									
Summarization of Prior Knowledge			Data Aggregation or Integration				Explanation Building		Critical Assessment of Extant Literature
Narrative Review	Descriptive Review	Scoping Review	Systematic Review	Meta-Analysis	Qualitative Meta-Synthesis	Umbrella Review	Theoretical Review	Realist Review	Critical Review
Types of Literature Reviews for Each Overarching Goal									

*Paré, Trudel, Jaana, and Kitsiou (2015)

Fig. 3.2 Typology* of literature reviews

- *Descriptive Review*: Reports the extent to which the sample of empirical studies supports or reveals any patterns or trends about preexisting propositions, theories, methodologies, or findings.
- *Scoping Review*: Provides an initial portrait of the literature on a specific topic. If the field of study is large, this is then a *Mapping Review*.

3.6.2 Goal: Data Aggregation or Integration

- *Systematic Review*: Uses a typical systematic review process, but in contrast to the meta-analytic approach uses narrative (not statistical) methods to describe the results of the included studies. If the health scholar urgently needs an answer to a research question, then this can be a *Rapid Review*.
- *Meta-analysis*: Uses statistical methods to aggregate quantitative data based on effect sizes from multiple studies mostly to describe the overall effect of an intervention.
- *Qualitative meta-synthesis*: Provides a systematic review and integration of findings from qualitative studies.
- *Umbrella Review*: Provides integration of evidence from multiple systematic reviews.

3.6.3 Goal: Explanation Building

- *Theoretical Review*: Uses conceptual and empirical studies to synthesize the literature into a theoretical overview and conceptual framework with proposed claims or hypotheses.
- *Realist Review*: Synthesizes prior studies to explain the mechanism of how complex interventions work (or why they fail) in contexts or settings. Realist reviews have no preference for either quantitative or qualitative evidence. They consider multiple methods to be valuable for the exploration of the processes and impacts of complex interventions.

3.6.4 Goal: Critical Assessment of Extant Literature

- *Critical Review*: Provides a critical analysis of the extant (existing) literature on a broad topic to reveal weaknesses, contradictions, controversies, or inconsistencies.

Table 3.4 offers additional information that can assist the health scholar in deciding the best type of literature review to carry out for a specific purpose and a specific

Table 3.4 Literature review sources and analysis

	Sources		Analysis	
Type of review[a]	Conceptual sources	Empirical sources	Quantitative analysis	Qualitative analysis
Narrative review	Yes	Yes		Narrative summary
Descriptive review		Yes	Frequency analysis	Content analysis
Scoping or mapping review	Yes	Yes	Frequency analysis	Content analysis
Systematic review or rapid review		Yes (quantitative)		Narrative synthesis
Meta-analysis		Yes	Meta-analysis	
Qualitative meta-synthesis		Yes (qualitative)		Narrative synthesis
Umbrella review		Systematic reviews		Narrative synthesis
Theoretical review	Yes	Yes		Content analysis and interpretive methods
Realist review		Yes (quantitative and qualitative)	Mixed-methods approach	
Critical review	Yes	Yes		Content analysis and critical interpretive methods

[a]Based on Paré et al. (2015)

review question. Although the review typology of Fig. 3.2 and Table 3.4 is extensive and covers many types of literature reviews, it is not comprehensive of all the types of published literature reviews. Reviews may have different names yet refer to the same thing. For example, some authors called a narrative review a résumé or empirical review, and a theoretical review may be called a synopsis review [8].

3.7 Semantics: Reviewing the Literature vs. A Literature Review

Clarifying the difference between conducting literature reviews and reviewing the literature is an important point. Reviewing the literature takes place when a scholar prepares the introductory section of any scholarly academic writing such as journal articles, including review articles. Reviewing the literature involves selectively discussing the literature on a particular topic to make the argument that a new study will make a new and/or important contribution to knowledge [9].

In contrast, conducting literature reviews is carrying out a type of research that has its distinct research design and methodology [10]. Rather than selectively reviewing relevant literature to make an argument about the need for a certain study, literature reviews provide a comprehensive synthesis of the available evidence to present the readers with conclusions about a body of work or a collection of studies.

There are several types of literature reviews including narrative, descriptive, scoping, meta-analytic, systematic, and others. They can be used to [8]:

- Summarize prior knowledge
- Aggregate and integrate data from different studies
- Build an explanation
- Critically assess the literature

3.7.1 Reviewing the Literature

For a review of the literature such as you would do in the introduction section of a manuscript, you want to be sure that you have a good grasp of the current state of the literature so you can feel confident providing a brief review at the start of your introduction. As each paragraph of your manuscript unfolds, you will want to build on your ideas with more evidence. This building should be smooth and gradual, so any conclusions flow naturally.

The introduction section should include the reasoning for selecting a guiding theory or framework for the educational project. The Discussion/Conclusion sections address how the results demonstrate the impact of the intervention in the context of the conceptual framework [2]. However, these sections of the manuscript are more than summaries of facts. The language of the manuscript introduction should be crafted thoughtfully to accurately inform the reader and to motivate and persuade the reader to understand the viewpoint of the writer. A good writer will make it compelling. It might help to think of the manuscript as a story [11], where the introduction section is an opportunity to tell the story of a problem and why it matters (or a gap in knowledge and why it matters). The Discussion/Conclusion sections are then used to tell how your piece adds to the story, what lessons come from the story you told, and what is the story-in-waiting. The chapter in this book on writing will discuss these ideas in more detail.

3.7.2 The Scoping Review

Scoping reviews have seen a noticeable increase in publishing. One reason might be that the methodological framework for completing such a review was published by Arksey and O'Malley [12] and by Levac et al. [13]. Another might be that scholars have found scoping reviews to be a convenient methodology that provides a good balance between effort and returns on investment. Conducting a scoping review does not require the same amount of effort and resources that a systematic review or meta-analysis requires, yet the review gives a useful quality appraisal, can answer important questions, and has the potential to be published in a reputable journal. Additionally, the learning curve is less steep for doing a scoping review compared with other types of reviews. The Appendix of this book provides additional details for the steps in conducting a scoping review.

3.8 The Annotated Bibliography as a Starting Point

An annotated bibliography is a useful tool that can help in the literature review process. In an annotated bibliography, a short paragraph or two is written for each reference you find in the literature that you think is important for your work. For example, you might start a document named "Annotated Bibliography for Scholarly Project." In it, you would put the citation for any articles you think are relevant. When you read the articles, write two paragraphs, one with a brief summary of the article and one that answers the question, "How does this article relate to my project?" You might find that some articles do not relate very well. Others do relate and will later be useful when you are putting thoughts together for the introduction or discussion section of your manuscript.

The annotated bibliography can also be used to help with the following
1. Provide a summary of each source: The brief summaries in an annotated bibliography provide a quick overview of each source's content, scope, and relevance to your research. This helps you to quickly determine whether and how a source might be useful for your research.
2. Provide an evaluation of each source: The comments and annotations that you write in an annotated bibliography can help you evaluate the quality of the source when you critically examine each source and write your notes about it.

3.9 Conclusion

A health scholar must first grasp what exists in the literature before producing scholarship. A good understanding of the literature is needed to set boundaries, provide a context, show trends, or identify problems and gaps. Research gaps can be categorized into five types—overlooked (a gap in the current state of research), extension based (a gap for extending and complementing existing literature), needing empirical support (an area with a lack of empirical support), under-researched (not received enough attention and investigation), and confusion (research with competing explanations). Different types of literature reviews are used for different purposes. When first starting a scholarly project, it might be helpful to keep track of articles that you feel might be applicable with an annotated bibliography.

3.10   Questions

Activities

1. Find three articles that relate to your area of interest. For each article, write two paragraphs.

    (a) Label the first paragraph for each article, "Summary," and write 2–4 sentences that summarize the article contents.

    (b) Label the second paragraph for each article, "How does this article relate to my project." Write 3–4 sentences about how the article is directly helpful to your project.

    - For example, an article might help by giving you an insight on data collection methods, or it might help in explaining an obstacle the study team encountered and how they overcame it.

References

1. Boote DN, Beile P. Scholars before researchers: on the centrality of the dissertation literature review in research preparation. Educ Res. 2005;34(6):3–15. https://doi.org/10.3102/0013189X034006003.
2. Zackoff MW, Real FJ, Abramson EL, Li STT, Klein MD, Gusic ME. Enhancing educational scholarship through conceptual frameworks: a challenge and roadmap for medical educators. Acad Pediatr. 2019;19(2):135–41.
3. Pickering C, Byrne J. The benefits of publishing systematic quantitative literature reviews for PhD candidates and other early-career researchers. Higher Educ Res Dev. 2014;33(3):534–48. https://doi.org/10.1080/07294360.2013.841651.
4. Varpio L, Paradis E, Uijtdehaage S, Young M. The distinctions between theory, theoretical framework, and conceptual framework. Acad Med. 2020;95(7):989–94.
5. Creswell JW, Guetterman TC. Educational research: planning, conducting, and evaluating quantitative and qualitative research. 6th ed. New York: Pearson; 2019.
6. Sandberg J, Alvesson M. Ways of constructing research questions: gap-spotting or problematization? Organization. 2011;18(1):23–44. https://doi.org/10.1177/1350508410372151.
7. Lingard L. Writing an effective literature review Part I: mapping the gap. Perspect Med Educ. 2018;7(1):47–9. https://doi.org/10.1007/s40037-017-0401-x.
8. Paré G, Trudel MC, Jaana M, Kitsiou S. Synthesizing information systems knowledge: A typology of literature reviews. Information & Management. 2015;52(2):183–99.
9. Siddaway AP, Wood AM, Hedges LV. How to do a systematic review: a best practice guide for conducting and reporting narrative reviews, meta-analyses, and meta-syntheses. Annu Rev Psychol. 2019;70:747–70. https://doi.org/10.1146/annurev-psych-010418-102803.
10. Snyder H. Literature review as a research methodology: an overview and guidelines. J Bus Res. 2019;104(2019):333–9. https://doi.org/10.1016/j.jbusres.2019.07.039.
11. Lingard L, Watling C. It's a story not a study: writing an effective research paper academic medicine. 2016;91(12):e12. https://doi.org/10.1097/ACM.0000000000001389.
12. Arksey H, O'Malley L. Scoping studies: towards a methodological framework. Int J Soc Res Methodol. 2005;8(1):19–32. https://doi.org/10.1080/1364557032000119616.
13. Levac D, Colquhoun H, O'Brien KK. Scoping studies: advancing the methodology. Implementation science. 2010;5:1–9.

Chapter 4
Designing a Research Question

Ahmed Ibrahim and Camille L. Bryant

4.1 Introduction

Research questions are vital to qualitative, quantitative, and mixed-methods research. They "narrow the research objective and research purpose" ([1]: p 475; [2, 3]) and determine the study methods (e.g., research paradigm, design, sampling method, instruments, and analysis). Despite the essential role the question holds in guiding and focusing research, White [4] noted that academic literature and texts often neglect its importance for new scholars. Designing good research questions is part of designing a good study. It must be based on sound literature, investigate an important topic, and be focused on a critical gap that is related to an important problem that needs to be solved. With respect to the latter, research questions can address a problem related to gaps in the literature or contextual problems gleaned from applied practice [3]. This chapter starts with an overview of different types of questions in research and then considers how to discuss your research questions with other scholars.

Sharing your research question with the academic community is like joining a conversation at a social gathering, "you join the conversation with a contribution that signals your shared interest in the topic, your knowledge of what's already been said, and your intention to add something new that will matter to those participating" ([5]: p 252). When one does not follow this metaphorical protocol of joining a conversation, "backs turn or eyes roll, or both", which is the equivalent of being rejected or judged to be unworthy of joining the conversation. This chapter will help scholars learn how to join the conversation of scholars by designing a research question and sharing it.

A. Ibrahim (✉) · C. L. Bryant
Johns Hopkins University School of Education, Baltimore, MD, USA
e-mail: aibrahim@jhu.edu

A. S. Fitzgerald, G. Bosch (eds.), *Education Scholarship in Healthcare*,
https://doi.org/10.1007/978-3-031-38534-6_4

4.2 Types of Research Questions

Research questions are best designed and then developed when they are problem based and/or address a specific gap in a body of literature from its focused topics and subtopics. Generally speaking, research questions fall into three categories—descriptive, predictive, and causal—although more sophisticated systems of classifying research questions exist [6–9].

These three question types are not limited to educational research; they are generalizable to all empirical research fields. Description, prediction, and explanation (e.g., causality) are the goals of the scientific method [10]. The same is true in health settings; see Table 4.1.

Descriptive questions are used to "define, classify, catalog, or categorize events" ([10]: p 40). The main objective is to measure (quantify) a construct (quantitative research) or describe (qualify) a phenomenon (qualitative research).

Predictive questions are used to foretell the value of a variable or the occurrence of an event in the future, based on another variable or a set of variables. The main objective is to be able to estimate the value or occurrence of events with some precision. Predictive questions rely on correlations and regressions as tools and methods to relate variables that covary (vary together) and estimate relations among them.

Table 4.1 Three types of research questions

Research questions	Objectives	Type of research	Examples
Descriptive	Properties and nonexperimental comparisons (equivalences and differences)	Qualitative descriptive	The hidden curriculum of medical/nursing school
		Quantitative descriptive	Prevalence of bullying on the wards
		Mixed-methods descriptive	Curriculum and application in practice
Predictive	Relations and correlations	Correlational	Predictive performance on exams
		Mixed-methods correlational	Predictive behavioral outcomes and observations
Causal	Conditionality and causality	Quasi-experimental and experimental	Curriculum effectiveness
		Mixed-methods causal comparative, quasi-experimental, and experimental	Training effectiveness and barriers

Causal questions are used to address (in an explanatory way) the effect of one or more variables on another variable. The main objective is to be able to establish a link between a *cause* and *effect*. Causal questions ask about the effect or influence of a variable representing a construct or an intervention on an outcome or a number of outcomes. It is critical to be careful about the language used in expressing research questions asking about causal effects. Many new scholars confuse the terms or language used and ask questions about effects while thinking about correlational predictive studies. The objective of causal questions is to establish causality.

4.3 Characteristics of Quality Research Questions

Quality research questions align with the research problem and purpose [11]. In addition, they are written clearly to reduce any ambiguity. Specificity regarding the participants, context, and constructs explored are also important characteristics to consider when writing research questions. Finally, questions should also be answerable and meaningful.

4.4 Quantitative Research Questions: The PICO Framework

For quantitative questions, a framework known as *PICO* is helpful. PICO is an acronym—*Population/Participants (P), Intervention/Independent Variable (I), Comparison (C), and Outcomes (O)*. Using these components to form a question helps ensure that the question is clear and answerable. The PICO framework can be modified and adapted to suit the different types of quantitative research questions; see Table 4.2.

4.4.1 Quantitative Descriptive Questions: P–O Framework

In quantitative descriptive questions, the PICO framework is modified to PO (*Population/Participants* and *Outcomes*) since there is no independent variable (I) that is manipulated, and no comparison groups (C) are used. For example, a question can be formulated as "What is the (outcome) of (participants) on (descriptor)?"

Table 4.2 Research questions frameworks and examples using ABIM/examinees

Questions	Framework	Generic template	Example
Descriptive quantitative	P–O	**What is the** *outcome* **of** *participants* **on** *descriptor*?	**What is the** *distribution of scores* **for** internal medicine *examinees* **on** *the ABIM recertification exam*?
Predictive quantitative	PI-O	**Does** *intervention* **affect** *outcome* **in** *population/participant*?	**Does** *taking a review course* **affect** *the ABIM exam pass rate* **in** *recertification examinees*?
Causal quantitative	PICO	**Does** *intervention* **have** *outcome* **on** *population/participant* **compared with** *comparison group*?	**Does** *maintenance of certification participation* **lead to** *higher scores on recertification testing* **for** internal medicine *examinees* **compared to** *those who do not participate*?
	PICOT	**In** *population,* **does** *intervention* **compared with** *control* **cause** *outcome* **within** *timeframe*?	**In** internal medicine *examinees,* **does** *a review course* **compared with** *independent study* **affect** *the pass rate on the ABIM exam* **when** *the review course is within 6 months of the exam*?
Qualitative	PPhTS	**For** *participants,* **what is their** *central phenomenon,* **during** *time* **in** *space*?	**For** *ABIM recertification examinees,* **what is their** *perception of overall burden of testing* **during** *their most recent test experience* **in** *the new home format*?

P population/participants, *I* intervention/independent, *V* variable, *C* comparison, *O* outcomes, *T* time, *Ph* phenomenon, *S* space

4.4.2 Quantitative Predictive Questions: PI-O Framework

In quantitative predictive (correlational) questions, the PICO framework is modified to PIO (*Population/Participant, Intervention/Independent* Variables, and *Outcomes*) since there are no comparison groups (C). For example, a question can be formulated as "Does (intervention) influence (outcome) in (population/participant)?"

4.4.3 Quantitative Causal Questions: PICO Framework

In quantitative causal questions, the full PICO framework can be used (*Population/Participants, Intervention/Independent* Variable, *Comparison,* and *Outcomes*). For example, a question can be formulated as "Does (intervention) have (outcome) on (population/participant) compared with (comparison group)?" All four components of the PICO question are used.

If participants are randomized and assigned to either the intervention or the comparison group, then there is causality based on the results. The causality can be relative to the comparison group, a manipulation in the way all participants in each group are exposed to an intervention, and/or temporal ordering because the populations get the interventions at different times.

4.4.4 Quantitative Effect Over Time: PICOT Framework

When you are interested in looking at the effect of an intervention over a particular period of time, the variable for *time (T)* is included in the question framing, and the framework becomes PICOT (*Population/Participants, Intervention/Independent* Variable, *Comparison,* and *Outcomes, Time*). For example, the question can be formulated as "In (population), does (intervention) compared with (control) cause (outcome) within (timeframe)?"

4.5 Qualitative Research Questions: The PPhTS Framework

The purpose of qualitative research is to ask questions that lead to describing a central phenomenon that may take place within a qualitative case or culture. The central phenomenon is defined as "the concept or a process explored in qualitative research" [12]. A phenomenon can be a story (narrative), a lived experience (phenomenology), a theory (grounded theory), a culture (ethnography), or a case or multiple cases (case study).

For qualitative questions, four essential components should be addressed to ensure that the question is clear and answerable. We propose calling this framework the *PPhTS* framework. PPhTS is an acronym for *Participants, central Phenomenon, Time, and Space (i.e., context)*. For example, using the PPhTS framework, a qualitative question can be formulated as "For (Participants), what is their (central Phenomenon), during (Time) in (Space)?"

Note that qualitative research uses *"what"* for the description of processes and *"how"* for mechanisms or processes (rather than *why,* which is causality) to ask questions.

4.5.1 Qualitative Questions Often Evolve and Change

In designing qualitative research questions, the health scholar should be aware that the qualitative question often matures over time with the study itself. This change signals growth and depth of understanding and should be welcomed and not feared [12]. Qualitative questions not only change and emerge during the study but also evolve as one is studying the phenomenon [13]. As Agee [14] puts it, "conceptualizing, developing, writing, and re-writing research questions are all part of a dynamic, reflective qualitative inquiry process".

4.6 Mixed-Methods Research Questions

Mixed methods are used if integrating both quantitative and qualitative research approaches would provide a deeper understanding of a phenomenon along with strong evidence for description, association, or causality [1, 11, 15]. Mixed-methods questions are unique in that qualitative and quantitative research questions can be separated or combined into one question [16]. As such, PICO and PPhTS frameworks can be used together to formulate mixed-methods questions. Combining the question frameworks allows the scholar to provide a strong description and explanation of the research situation. Further, like qualitative research questions, mixed-methods questions may evolve throughout the study [1].

4.7 Presenting the Research Question: The CARS Model

In the metaphor of joining a conversation in a well-structured manner, a research question needs to emerge from knowledge of work that has come in the field prior. The *Create A Research Space (CARS)* model [17, 18] is a way to introduce a research question to others such as in an academic setting or article. It consists of

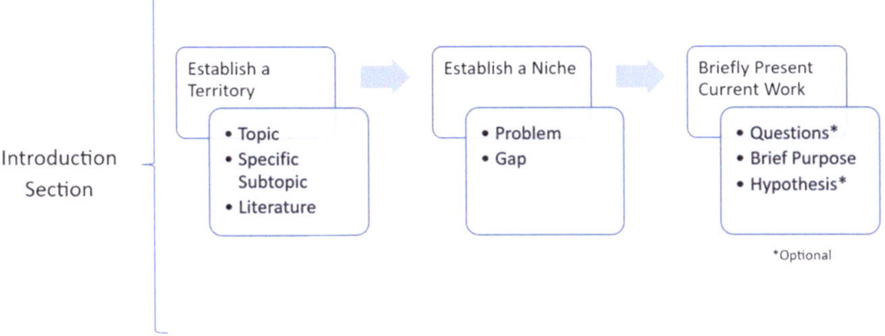

Fig. 4.1 The logical moves and steps of introducing research questions

three parts called "moves"—establish the literature territory, establish a niche, and then describe the purpose of the research (Fig. 4.1).

4.7.1   Move 1: Establish Literary Territory—Anchoring a Topic in Literature

In this first step or "move" of the CARS model, the scholar sets the context of research that has come before and provides the necessary background on the topic to be studied. This is done by introducing a topic, discussing a specific subtopic, and anchoring the topic and subtopic in the existing literature.

When introducing the topic, the health scholar should start with the broad subject matter. The reason to do this is to make an appeal to those who might not be familiar with the topic in question but may have related interests or knowledge. Several tactics are used to engage others such as [19]:

- Rhetorical questions
- Relating the topic to everyday experiences
- Analogies and metaphors
- Statistics or facts
- Historical references

The scholar then makes moves from the broad generalizations to the specifics surrounding current knowledge, practices, or phenomena in the field [18], from *uncontentious generalizations* ([20]: p 94) to *knowledge claims*. Lingard [21] defines knowledge claims as "a way of presenting the growing understanding of the community of researchers who have been exploring your topic."

By anchoring the topic and subtopic in the literature, the health scholar relates the knowledge claims and topic generalizations to the literature. It is important to cite both seminal works in the literature and recent works. Citing both shows that you have a good command of the field, its history, context, and recent developments.

4.7.2   Move 2: Establish a Niche—The Problem and Gap

The second move in the CARS model is to establish a niche, which is a gap in the existing research or a deficiency in the current state of knowledge that needs to be filled through additional research.

- In *identifying a problem*, the researcher describes an issue or a concern that people are talking about. The problem could be practical and arise from experience and supported by sources from the literature and could be theoretical, arising from the discovery of an anomaly or dissonance in studies.
- In *establishing a gap*, the researcher describes something that is missing in research and that needs to be solved to attain a better state of understanding or a solution to a problem.

4.7.3   Move 3: Occupy the Niche—Purpose, Question, Quantitative Hypothesis

The third move in the CARS model is to occupy the niche [17] or present the current work [18]. The main requirement in this move is to announce the present research descriptively. According to the CARS model, presenting a research question or hypothesis is optional. It can be understood that presenting a research question is optional because descriptively presenting the current work could show the intent of the work. Additionally, the research question can be a restatement of the purpose in an interrogative way. However, presenting the research questions can accomplish more than what the purpose statement could. The research questions can be numerous and specific. They also connect to methods, results, and conclusions in one-to-one correspondences.

In *presenting the purpose*, the scholar states the focus of the research ([12]: p 110). A straightforward statement can be used: "The purpose of this research is …."

In *stating the research question*, the author asks the question that motivated the research.

In *stating the hypotheses for quantitative research*, the author presents statements that provide a prediction that is informed by prior research. Hypotheses are defined as "statements in quantitative research in which the investigator makes a prediction or a conjecture about the outcome of a relationship among attributes or characteristics" ([12]: p 110). The CARS model illustrates the important connections between the research problem, research purpose, and subsequent hypothesis (quantitative research), all of which must align with the research question(s).

4.8 Conclusion

Developing quality research questions is a skill that requires practice. The PICO and PPhTS frameworks help scholars develop research questions for a variety of research purposes across the three research paradigms. The generic template for each question type is especially useful for novice researchers who are new to developing research questions. These templates provide a model for writing quantitative, qualitative, and mixed-methods research questions for descriptive, correlational, or causal studies. Using this guide, the health scholar can write purposeful questions that align with the research problem and objective and are specific and answerable. These characteristics are critical as the research questions are the pathway to making methodological decisions to conduct the study.

4.9 Questions

Activities
1. Who will be the population/participants (P) for your project?
2. If you plan to do a quantitative project, list which of the following apply to your project (note: your project might not have all the following):

   (a) Intervention/independent variable (I)
   (b) Comparison (C)
   (c) Outcome (O)

3. If you plan to do a qualitative project, list which of the following apply to your project (note: your project might not have all the following):

   (a) Time (T)
   (b) Phenomenon (Ph)
   (c) Space (S)

4. State your question using the appropriate framework, PICO or PPhTS.

References

1. Onwuegbuzie A, Leech N. Linking research questions to mixed methods data analysis procedures 1. Qual Rep. 2006;11(3):474–98. https://doi.org/10.46743/2160-3715/2006.1663.
2. Creswell JW, Poth CN. Qualitative inquiry and research design: choosing among five approaches. 4th ed. Thousand Oaks: Sage; 2018.
3. Johnson B, Christensen LB. Educational research: quantitative, qualitative, and mixed approaches. Thousand Oaks: Sage Publications, Inc.; 2020.

4. White P. Who's afraid of research questions? The neglect of research questions in the methods literature and a call for question-led methods teaching. Int J Res Method Educ. 2013;36(3):213–27. https://doi.org/10.1080/1743727x.2013.809413.

5. Lingard L. Joining a conversation: the problem/gap/hook heuristic. Perspect Med Educ. 2015;4(5):252–3. https://doi.org/10.1007/s40037-015-0211-y.

6. Dillon JT. The classification of research questions. Rev Educ Res. 1984;54(3):327–61. https://doi.org/10.3102/00346543054003327.

7. Dillon JT. Finding the question for evaluation research. Stud Educ Eval. 1987;13(2):139–51. https://doi.org/10.1016/S0191-491X(87)80027-5.

8. Smith NL. Toward the justification of claims in evaluation research. Eval Program Plann. 1987;10(4):309–14. https://doi.org/10.1016/0149-7189(87)90002-4.

9. Smith NL, Mukherjee P. Classifying research questions addressed in published evaluation studies. Educ Eval Policy Anal. 1994;16(2):223–30. https://doi.org/10.3102/01623737016002223.

10. Shaughnessy JJ, Zechmeister EB, Zechmeister JS. Research methods in psychology. 9th ed. New York: McGraw Hill; 2011.

11. DeCuir-Gunby JT, Schutz PA. Developing a mixed methods proposal a practical guide for beginning researchers. Thousand Oaks: Sage; 2017.

12. Creswell JW, Guetterman TC. Educational research: planning, conducting, and evaluating quantitative and qualitative research. 6th ed. New York: Pearson; 2019.

13. Ely M, Anzul M, Friedman T, Ganer D, Steinmetz AM. Doing qualitative research: circles within circles. London: Falmer Press; 1991.

14. Agee J. Developing qualitative research questions: a reflective process. Int J Qual Stud Educ. 2009;22(4):431–47. https://doi.org/10.1080/09518390902736512.

15. Johnson RB, Onwuegbuzie AJ. Mixed methods research: a research paradigm whose time has come. Educ Res. 2004;33(7):14–26. https://doi.org/10.3102/0013189x033007014.

16. Creamer EG. An introduction to fully integrated mixed methods research. Thousand Oaks: Sage; 2018.

17. Swales J. Genre analysis: English in academic and research settings. Cambridge: Cambridge University Press; 1990.

18. Swales J. Research genres: explorations and applications. Cambridge: Cambridge University Press; 2004.

19. Kendall PC, Norris LA, Rifkin LS, Silk JS. Introducing your research report: writing the introduction. In: Sternberg RJ, editor. Guide to publishing in psychology journals. 2nd ed. Cambridge: Cambridge University Press; 2018. p. 37–53. https://doi.org/10.1017/9781108304443.005.

20. Thomson P, Kamler B. Writing for peer reviewed journals: strategies of getting published. Abingdon: Routledge; 2013.

21. Lingard L. Writing an effective literature review: Part I: Mapping the gap. Perspectives on Medical Education. 2018;7:47–49.

Chapter 5
Research Methods

Camille L. Bryant

5.1 Introduction: The Three Research Paradigms

To address research questions and satisfy the purpose of research, it is important to understand research paradigms. "A research paradigm is a perspective, about research held by a community of researchers that is based on a set of shared assumptions, concepts, values, and practices" ([1]: p 31). There are three research paradigms—quantitative, qualitative, and mixed methods. In this chapter, each paradigm is discussed with respect to their general characteristics, including data types, philosophical stances (i.e., the ways of knowing), sampling, and data analysis approaches.

Quantitative research relies on numerical data and is rooted in the positivist and postpositivist philosophical stances [2] in which phenomena are explored to ascertain a singular truth (Table 5.1). As such, objectivity is essential—the researcher, and their inherent biases, cannot interfere in the empirical examination of phenomena. Further, findings should generalize across time and context [3]. Therefore, knowledge is determined from causal inferences, exploration of key variables, measurement, and theory testing [2].

Qualitative research explores nonnumerical data such as words from interviews, focus groups, and observation. Qualitative data also includes data from pictures and drawings. This research paradigm is rooted in the philosophical stances of constructivism, relativism, and idealism, to name a few. Here, the notion of a singular truth is replaced by the idea that multiple realities exist. Further, the role of the researcher is central to the understanding of phenomena. Thus, subjectivity is an embedded characteristic of qualitative research.

Mixed-methods research is the third research paradigm [4] and relies on numerical and nonnumerical data. As such, a researcher uses quantitative and qualitative

C. L. Bryant (✉)
Johns Hopkins University School of Education, Baltimore, MD, USA
e-mail: cbryan16@jhu.edu

A. S. Fitzgerald, G. Bosch (eds.), *Education Scholarship in Healthcare*,
https://doi.org/10.1007/978-3-031-38534-6_5

Table 5.1 Philosophical assumptions of quantitative, qualitative, and mixed-methods research

	Positivist	Postpositivist	Constructivist	Transformative	Pragmatism
Research paradigm(s)	Quantitative	Quantitative mixed methods	Qualitative mixed methods	Mixed methods	Mixed methods

data to satisfy the research purpose and examine the research questions. The strength of mixed-methods research is that it allows the researcher to maximize the strengths and minimize the weaknesses of the quantitative and qualitative research paradigms (p 15). Mixed-methods research is rooted in the postpositivist, constructivist, transformative, and the more popular pragmatic philosophical stances [2].

5.2 Variables in Social Science Research

A *variable* is any entity that can vary by taking on multiple values. A *latent* variable in quantitative research is a type of variable that is not directly measured or observed. In this case, you rely on indicators to measure or observe the variable. For example, health is a construct. It is indirectly measured by examining one's BMI, blood pressure, blood sugar, etc.

Quantitative variables can *be discrete* or *continuous.*

- A *discrete* variable is a variable that can be counted in whole units such as the number of patients.
- A *continuous* variable is one that has an infinite number of values between two values such as weight.

5.3 Quantitative Research

Quantitative research answers questions that generally aim to understand the extent of change that one or more variables cause on an outcome(s), or the influence that one or more variables have on others. These questions are answered using experimental and nonexperimental research methods.

Experimental Research Experimental research examines causal relationships. The researcher is interested in knowing if x causes b. An example is a study to determine if exposure to a text messaging intervention on COVID-19 vaccine reminders increases the number of fully vaccinated participants who have received one of two doses of the vaccine. The group who received the text messages are called the *experimental group.* To determine if the intervention caused increases in the full vaccination rate, there must be a comparison group. In experimental research, this comparison group that does not receive the intervention is called the *control group.* Experimental research relies on the manipulation of groups, as the researcher has designed a scenario in which one group receives text messages and the other does not. This manipulated variable is called the *independent variable*. In this example, we might call the independent variable, text message status, where one group receives text messages, and the other group does not. The researcher aims to determine if the manipulation of text messaging status affects the outcome of full vaccination rates. This outcome is regarded as the *dependent variable*.

While this seems simple enough, social science research does not operate in a controlled environment. Human beings are not in labs and devoid of experiences and influence. As such, the researcher must account for *confounding* or *extraneous variables* that may influence the outcome but are not under investigation. These terms are often used interchangeably and are important to consider. A confounding variable from the vaccine text messaging study might be personal influences such as family members who encourage the second dose, ads on vaccination, and intrinsic responsibility. One way to mitigate extraneous factors is through the study design, particularly the sampling approach. By randomly sampling and assigning individuals to the treatment and control groups, the researcher can equalize the characteristics of the groups such that individuals in both groups are likely to experience the same types of influences on their behavior (in this case to receive their second dose). When this is the case, the researcher is better able to attribute any effects to the text messaging intervention and not the confounding factors.

It is important to note that while experimental research was discussed with respect to a control group and one treatment group, multiple treatment groups are common. Treatment conditions can vary in levels of exposure and type. For example, with respect to the text messaging intervention for second-dose COVID-19 vaccination reminders, one treatment group may receive two messages a week, while the other receives four messages a week. In this way, the levels of exposure vary across treatment conditions. Another study might include an e-mail reminder group in addition to the text messaging group. In this way, the type of treatment varies across groups.

Nonexperimental Research Nonexperimental research does not aim to examine causal relationships using manipulated variables. Instead, it examines the degree to which variables relate to one another. For example, a researcher interested in examining the relationship between medical students' self-efficacy (i.e., belief in their ability to deliver patient-centered care) and patient-centered care attitudes [5] would rely on nonexperimental research. Nonexperimental research includes correlation and regression. Correlation and regression aim to understand how variables "move" together. When considering correlation using the variables mentioned (i.e., self-efficacy and patient-centered care attitudes), one essentially aims to know if: 1) patient-centered care attitudes increase as self-efficacy increases and therefore indicate a *positive relationship*, 2) patient-centered care attitudes decrease when self-efficacy increases, indicating a *negative or inverse relationship*, or 3) there is *no relationship* between patient-centered care attitudes and self-efficacy toward patient-centered care. Regression allows researchers to make predictions. Just as with experimental research, there is an independent and dependent variable. However, in this case, the researcher does not designate two or more groups for the independent variable. Instead, the independent variable for regression is one that influences the dependent variable. Here, the researcher may be interested in determining the degree to which medical students' self-efficacy (independent variable) influences/predicts patient-centered care attitudes (dependent variable). In other words, to what degree do patient-centered care attitudes change as self-efficacy changes or stated differently, what is the degree of change in attitudes given a unit change in self-efficacy?

5.3.1 Sampling

Sampling is the process through which researchers draw participants from the larger population. Samples should represent the sample such that the characteristics of the population are represented with the same proportions within the sample. This helps to reduce bias within the sample. Quantitative samples can be random or nonrandom. Random sampling is the process where participants are randomly chosen from the population. This is a more rigorous approach than nonrandom sampling, where participants are not randomly chosen from the population. Table 5.2 delineates the various random and nonrandom sampling approaches.

5.3.2 Validity and Reliability

When conducting quantitative research, ensuring that data are valid and reliable is important. There are two areas that must be considered when discussing validity and reliability; one deals with the findings of the research study directly, while the other deals with instrumentation. In thinking about the findings of the research study, *reliability* indicates that, if replicated, the findings of the study would remain consistent. *Validity* indicates that the results are valid or accurate such that the findings of the

Table 5.2 Types of sampling

Random sampling approaches		Nonrandom sampling approaches	
Simple random	Every person in the population has an equal chance of selection	Purposive	Individuals with certain characteristics are targeted
Stratified random	First, the population is grouped by strata. Second, participants are randomly chosen from each stratum	Convenience	Individuals who can be recruited easily are available and volunteers are chosen to participate
Systematic	First, an interval is chosen followed by randomly selecting a starting point between 1 and n; next, every nth person is selected for the study	Quota	First, the researcher determines the sample size for groups within the population and, second, conveniently samples from those groups
Cluster	First, clusters are established from the population; second, clusters are randomly selected	Snowball	Each person is asked to identify additional participants for the study

sample represent the larger population (*external validity*) and that the findings are due to the study intervention and not confounding factors (*internal validity*). Studies that are valid and reliable have strong designs that minimize the influence of extraneous variables within the study. With respect to instrumentation, validity indicates that the instrument accurately measures the construct and reliability relates to the consistency of the results over several trials. For example, a reliable scale to measure weight would measure weight with little variation given that all things are equal (e.g., if you were to step on the scale three times in a row, a reliable scale should vary minimally). It should also accurately measure your weight (validity).

5.3.3 Designs

Choosing an appropriate design to answer the research questions and satisfy the research purpose is an essential aspect of research. There are several designs to choose from depending on the type of research question. These designs are organized by the type of quantitative research one conducts (experimental vs. nonexperimental).

In this chapter, the common quantitative research designs are discussed and include two experimental designs—pretest-posttest control group design and posttest-only control group design, two quasi-experimental designs—nonequivalent comparison group design and pretest-posttest design—and two nonexperimental designs—correlation and regression [6].

Experimental Research Designs Experimental research designs aim to examine the degree to which an independent variable affects a dependent variable. In other words, the researcher aims to cause changes in an outcome by manipulating the input. To do this, the researcher must aim to rule out confounding variables that might influence the outcomes through a strong research design. The pretest-posttest control design is one experimental design that minimizes confounding factors. In this design, participants are randomly assigned to a treatment and control condition. Prior to the introduction of the intervention, participants take a pretest. Next, the treatment (i.e., intervention) is introduced. Once the intervention is complete, participants take a posttest. This design helps to ensure that the intervention and control groups are "equal" prior to the intervention. One would not want one group to already have an advantage that might influence the outcomes as it would muddy the potential finding that the intervention did indeed change the dependent variable. The posttest-only control group design is similar to the latter, except, as you might guess, there is no pretest. As such, the opportunity to ensure that the intervention and control groups are equal prior to the intervention lies in trusting that random sampling and assignment did indeed create groups with similar characteristics.

Quasi-Experimental Research Designs The purpose of quasi-experimental designs is the same as experimental designs [6]. The goal is to determine if x caused

y. However, in quasi-experimental studies, although participants may be randomly sampled, they are not randomly assigned to a treatment and control condition. Random assignment to treatment and control conditions may not be feasible, particularly in social science research where naturally existing groups might prohibit this action. As such, the researcher may rely on matching to mitigate confounding factors due to the lack of random sampling. Matching helps to equalize the groups to mitigate variables related to the dependent variable. For example, a researcher conducting a study examining the use of a flipped classroom with first-year medical students on their engagement in their anatomy course may match based on experience with this instructional mode and MCAT score.

The nonequivalent comparison group design is similar to the pretest posttest control design, in which participants are given a pretest prior to the intervention. Once the intervention is complete, participants take the posttest, in this case, a questionnaire on engagement. The repeated measures design is one in which all participants are exposed to the intervention and are measured repeatedly over time. As such, prior to the introduction of the intervention, participants take one or more pretests to establish a baseline. Once the intervention is introduced, participants are measured again one or more times to determine if the intervention affected the dependent variable. In this way, participants serve as their own control.

What is tricky about experimental and quasi-experimental studies is that the same research question can be answered using a different design. Some of this comes down to feasibility and access. For example, if the researcher question asks, "To what extent does the flipped classroom instructional approach in the first-year anatomy class affect medical students' engagement in the classroom?", the institution may not approve participants taking a pretest and posttest to minimize any added stress to students' first year. However, when given the opportunity, an experimental study, in which participants are randomly selected and assigned to a group, is stronger than a quasi-experimental study as the former does a better job at ruling out confounding variables from the model.

Nonexperimental Research Designs Correlation and regression are used to examine relationships between variables. Correlation examines the relationship between two or more variables. A research question examined using correlation might ask, "What is the extent of the relationship between medical students' MCAT scores and step 1 of the USMLE?" Regression allows researchers to make predictions based on the relationship between variables. An example research question using regression might ask "What is the degree of influence of the MCAT scores on step 1 of the USMLE?" If the influence is statistically significant, the researcher can predict a USMLE score given an MCAT score.

5.3.4 Quantitative Research Analysis

Analysis begins with knowing your research question and the type of data you are using to answer that question. In social science research, conducting research using numerical data may include surveys and questionnaires, assessments, and standardized tests, to name a few. Data can take one of the four levels of measurement. The first is nominal data. Nominal data assigns a number as a label. For example, one might assign the following to racial groups where 1 = Caucasian, 2 = African American, and 3 = Asian. The labels can take on any value since no mathematical operations can be performed. The numbers are solely for the purpose of labeling and distinguishing groups. Ordinal quantitative data is ranked data. For example, an admissions committee may rank students for acceptance into their occupational therapy program. Those with the higher rankings are accepted into the program. Values on the interval scale of measurement have no true zero. In other words, zero is not the absence of that entity. For example, the Celsius and Fahrenheit scales are measured at the interval level as the temperature of zero does not mean the absence of temperature. However, mathematically, the distance between values is meaningful. Finally, the ratio level of measurement has a true zero such as weight, pulse rate, body temperature (Kelvin), and height.

Descriptive Statistics Descriptive statistics should be the first level of analysis for any quantitative study. The examination of the mean, median, mode, standard deviation, variation, range, frequency, and so forth provides an initial understanding of what the data are "telling you." This first step also helps to triage any mistakes due to data entry error. Descriptive statistics are also useful for understanding how data differ across groups and contexts (disaggregated).

Hypothesis Testing Hypothesis testing is an approach to statistical analysis that allows researchers to draw conclusions from sample statistics to the population. This is regarded as inferential statistics because the researcher makes inferences about the population from the sample. This is done by examining two competing hypotheses— the null and the alternative. Hypothesis testing is probability based. The goal is to determine if the likelihood of the event is what one is likely to observe in the population (not statistically significant) or if the likelihood of the event is rare (statistically significant). Mull these ideas over for a bit. If the likelihood of the event is what one would normally observe, then the findings are not out of the ordinary and thus non-significant. They are what one would expect by chance. However, if the findings reveal that the likelihood of the event is rare, then the findings are significant. The null hypothesis indicates that there is no effect, meaning that the findings are what one would likely observe the majority of the time. In other words, the likelihood of observing the event in the population is high or common and thus statistically non-significant. The alternative hypothesis indicates that there is an effect, meaning the likelihood of observing the event in the population is rare, and thus if that data reveals the occurrence of this event, it is statistically significant. In order to draw conclusions from hypothesis testing, it is important to discuss the notion of error.

As mentioned, there are two hypotheses when using inferential statistics—the null and alternative hypotheses. When drawing conclusions, one either rejects the null hypothesis (statistically significant) or fails to reject the null hypothesis (not statistically significant). Given that hypothesis testing is based on the probability of an event, any conclusion drawn is subject to error. There are two types of error, Type I (alpha) and Type II (beta). The alpha level is the probability of making a Type I error. In other words, it is the probability of rejecting the null hypothesis, when the null hypothesis is true. As such, when one concludes that the findings are statistically significant, and the null hypothesis is rejected, then there is a chance that this decision was made in error. This is Type I error. The alpha level is generally 5%, meaning when the null hypothesis is rejected, there is a 5% chance that this was done in error. Type II error is the probability of failing to reject the null hypothesis when it should be rejected. Prior to the analysis, the researcher determines the alpha level and compares this to the p value (probability that the null is true as determined by the statistical analyses) that is determined by the statistical analysis of data. If the p value is greater than alpha, then the researcher fails to reject the null hypothesis (nonsignificant). If the p value is less than or equal to the alpha level, then the researcher rejects the null hypothesis (statistically significant) (Table 5.3).

Parametric vs. Nonparametric Tests Findings from statistical tests used for hypothesis testing are only trustworthy, if assumptions required for the test are met. Some tests require that data are normally distributed; these are *parametric tests*. This means that the data are bell shaped where the frequency of scores is equally distributed around the mean. Tests used for data that are not normally distributed (e.g., skewed or rectangular) are *nonparametric*.

Differences Between Group Means Research questions that aim to determine if the means of groups differ are analyzed using parametric and nonparametric tests.

An *independent t-test* is an inferential parametric test that examines differences between the means of two independent groups for a single dependent variable (Table 5.4). The groups are independent because the scores between the groups are not correlated. For example, if the researcher asked "To what extent does empathy in the doctor-patient relationship differ between male and female residents?" the empathy scores between the two groups are unrelated. The nonparametric version of this test is the *Mann–Whitney U test*.

When scores are correlated between two groups, they are said to be *dependent*. A parametric, *dependent t-test* examines differences across two related scores such as pre- and post-scores. For example, if the researcher asked "To what degree does

Table 5.3 Hypothesis testing error rules

Null hypothesis is	True		False	
Reject the null hypothesis (statistically significant)	Type I error = α	Probability of rejecting the null hypothesis when it should **not** have been rejected (false positive)	Power = 1 $-\beta$	Probability of correctly rejecting the null hypothesis when it is false (true positive)
Fail to reject the null hypothesis (statistically nonsignificant)	$1 - \alpha$	Probability of failing to reject the null hypothesis when it should not be rejected (true negative)	Type II error = β	Probability of failing to reject the null hypothesis when it should have been rejected (false negative)

Table 5.4 Inferential statistics tests

Test	Description	Sample research question	Null hypothesis	Alternative hypothesis	Assumptions
Independent *t*-test	Parametric Examines mean differences between two independent groups on one dependent variable	Does empathy in the doctor-patient relationship differ between male and female residents?	There is no difference between the group means	[a]There is a difference between the group means	• Interval or ratio level of measurement • Independent observations • Normal distribution • Equal variances between groups
Dependent *t*-test	Parametric Examines mean differences between two dependent/related groups on one dependent variable	To what degree does empathy in patient care change between the first 2 years of the residency experience?	There is no difference between the mean differences	There is a difference between the mean differences	• Interval or ratio level of measurement • Dependent observations • Normal distribution
One-way ANOVA	Parametric Examines the mean difference for one independent variable with two or more groups on one dependent variable	Do first- through fifth-year surgical residents differ in their self-efficacy of using multidisciplinary care with breast cancer patients?	There is no difference between the group means	There is a difference between the group means	• Interval or ratio level of measurement • Independent observations • Normal distribution • Equal variances between groups

(continued)

Table 5.4 (continued)

Test	Description	Sample research question	Null hypothesis	Alternative hypothesis	Assumptions
One-way MANOVA	Parametric Examines the mean difference for one independent variable with two or more groups on two or more dependent variables	To what degree do first- through fifth-year surgical residents differ in their patient empathy and compassion for amputation surgery due to type 2 diabetes?	There is no difference between the groups on the combined dependent variables	There is difference between the groups on the combined dependent variables	• Interval or ratio level of measurement • Independent observations • Normal distribution • No univariate or multivariate outliers • Equal covariance/ variance matrices between groups • Dependent variables are moderately correlated
Repeated measures ANOVA	Parametric Examines mean differences between two or more time points on one dependent variable	What is the extent of change in empathy towards patients over a 3-year residency experience?	There is no mean difference between the time points	There is a mean difference between the time points	• Interval or ratio level of measurement • Dependent observations • Normal distribution • Sphericity- equal variances of all group differences

Table 5.4 (continued)

Test	Description	Sample research question	Null hypothesis	Alternative hypothesis	Assumptions
Repeated measures MANOVA	Parametric Examines mean differences between two or more time points on two or more dependent variables	What is the extent of change in empathy and compassion towards patients over a 3-year residency experience?	There is no difference between the dependent scores on the combined dependent variables	There is a difference between the dependent scores on the combined dependent variables	• Interval or ratio level of measurement • Dependent observations • Normal distribution • No univariate or multivariate outliers • Equal covariance/ variance matrices between groups • Dependent variables are moderately correlated
Factorial ANOVA	Parametric Examines mean differences for two or more independent variables each with two or more groups on one dependent variable	To what extent does sex and race influence the perceptions of nursing care within a suburban hospital?	There is no difference between the group means (for each independent variable) There is no interaction between the independent variables	There is a difference between the group means (for each independent variable) There is an interaction between the independent variables	• Interval or ratio level of measurement • Independent observations • Normal distribution • Equal variances between groups

(continued)

Table 5.4 (continued)

Test	Description	Sample research question	Null hypothesis	Alternative hypothesis	Assumptions
Factorial MANOVA	Parametric Examines mean differences for two or more independent variables each with two or more groups on two or more dependent variables	To what extent does sex and race influence the perceptions of empathy and nursing care within a suburban hospital?	There is no difference between the groups on the combined dependent variables There is no interaction between the independent variables on the combined dependent variables	There is difference between the groups on the combined dependent variables There is an interaction between the groups on the combined dependent variables	• Interval or ratio level of measurement • Independent observations • Normal distribution • No univariate or multivariate outliers • Equal covariance/variance matrices between groups • Dependent variables are moderately correlated
Pearson correlation	Parametric Examines the relationship between two variables	What is the relationship between the MCAT and USMLE step 1 scores?	There is not a relationship between the variables	There is a relationship between the variables	• Interval or ratio level of measurement • Normal distribution • Linear relationship between variables • Equal variances (spread of scores) around the regression line. This is called homoscedasticity

Table 5.4 (continued)

Test	Description	Sample research question	Null hypothesis	Alternative hypothesis	Assumptions
Spearman's rho correlation	Nonparametric Examines the relationship between two variables where one is at least ordinal/ranked	What is the relationship between podiatry school ranking (ordinal) and yearly salary (ratio) for podiatrists from historically marginalized populations?	There is not a relationship between the variables	There is a relationship between the variables	• Ordinal, interval or ratio level of measurement • The variables have a monotonic relationship such that as one variable increases, the other increases, or as one variable decreases, the other increases
Linear regression	Parametric Examines the influence of one variable on another for the purpose of prediction	What is the influence of research self-efficacy on the academic achievement of graduate students in a health profession?	The model coefficients are equal to zero	The model coefficients are not equal to zero	• Interval or ratio level of measurement • Normal distribution • Linear relationship between variables • Equal variances (spread of scores) around the regression line. This is called homoscedasticity

(continued)

Table 5.4 (continued)

Test	Description	Sample research question	Null hypothesis	Alternative hypothesis	Assumptions
Chi-square	Nonparametric Examines the association between nominal (categorical) variables	What is the association between admissions decisions and ethnicity for top-tier medical schools?	There is no association between the variables	There is an association between the variables	• Nominal level of measurement • Data contains frequency counts • Data are mutually exclusive—participants cannot be assigned to multiple category levels (e.g., someone reports that they have both been accepted and denied to Stanford during the same admission cycle)

[a]The alternative hypotheses can also be directional (e.g., the mean for group 1 is greater than the mean for group 2 or the mean for group 1 is less than the mean for group 2)

empathy in patient care change between the first two years of the residency experience?" the researcher might examine empathy scores of individuals at the beginning and end of residency. These scores are related because the same individuals are surveyed and their scores are correlated across the two time points. The nonparametric test to examine differences between dependent scores is the *Wilcoxon signed-rank test*.

The ANOVA test (sometimes called the *F*-test) examines differences on a single dependent variable between two or more groups. The one-way ANOVA has one independent variable with two or more levels (groups). For example, a researcher might ask, "To what degree do first-, second-, third-, fourth-, and fifth-year surgical residents differ in their self-efficacy of using multidisciplinary care with breast cancer patients?" In this case, the independent variable, year of surgical residency, has five levels or groups (first through fifth years). The ANOVA tests allow for multiple independent variables. When the researcher moves beyond one independent variable, they can employ a factorial ANOVA. If we expanded the research question to "To what degree does year of surgical residency and surgical specialty affect the self-efficacy of using multidisciplinary care with patients?" we would still have the independent variable with five levels (first through fifth years of surgical residency). The second independent variable is surgical specialty. This may have two levels where the groups are neurological and cardiothoracic surgery. This is called a 5×2 factorial ANOVA where 5 and 2 are the number of groups (levels) for each independent variable. The factorial model allows for the examination of three hypotheses simultaneously … differences between the means for each independent variable (main effects) and an interaction effect. An interaction examines differences between the combined independent variables. For example, a statistically significant interaction may demonstrate that self-efficacy for years 1–3 is statistically the same for both surgical specialties, but in years 4 and 5, cardiothoracic residents have statistically higher self-efficacy than neurological surgical residents. The pattern of self-efficacy across the 5 years varies depending on the surgical specialty.

Variations of the ANOVA include the repeated measures ANOVA, which examines mean differences over two or more time points (e.g., pre-mid-post); the split-plot factorial model, which examines mean difference between groups and across multiple time points; and the MANOVA test, which allows the researcher to examine differences between groups for multiple dependent variables. The MANOVA is similar to the ANOVA in that there can be one independent variable, multiple independent variables, and time points, the difference being that there are multiple dependent variables.

Correlation, Linear Regression, and Measure of Association Correlation and regression explore relationships between variables. These tests are not used to determine causation, but how variables influence one another. This relationship can be positive (both variables increase and decrease together) or negative/inverse (one variable increases while the other decreases). The r-value generated from a correlation analysis ranges from -1 to $+1$, where values closer to $+/- 1$ indicate stronger relationships, and values closer to 0 indicate weaker relationships. An r-value of $+/- 1$ is a perfect relationship. As with any inferential statistical test, certain assumptions must be met to trust the findings. These assumptions determine which type of correlational test is used such as the Pearson, Spearman's rho, etc.

Linear regression also examines relationships; however, one is able to make predictions using the equation for a line where Y (dependent variable+ $= B$ (slope of the independent variable) $x + c$ (y-intercept). More complex regression models include multiple regression where the influence of multiple independent variables on a dependent variable is examined and structural equational modeling which allows for the examination of relationships between latent variables.

Chi-square is a measure of association when examining the frequency of nominal variables. This test determines if nominal (categorical) variables are independent or associated. For example, if the researcher is interested in examining the association between white and non-white medical students' passage of the medical board, the researcher has two categorical variables. The first relates to racial status, white and non-white, while the second relates to board passage status, passed or failed. The frequency for each combined category (i.e., white and passed, non-white and passed, white and failed, non-white and failed) is examined to determine if passing or failing is associated with one's racial status. In other words, the researcher aims to determine if race matters when it comes to passing or failing boards. A statistically significant association would indicate that race does matter. The researcher can then examine the passage rates to determine how one group compares to the other.

5.3.5 *Effect Sizes*

Analysis of quantitative data using inferential statistics does not end with comparing the α-level to the p-value to determine statistical significance. Another statistic, the effect size, also provides valuable information. Effect sizes indicate how different mean scores are between groups in standard units (e.g., Cohen's d) or how much variation in the dependent variable is attributed to the independent variable (e.g., R^2) or mean differences (ω^2).

5.4 Qualitative Research

Qualitative research questions generally aim to understand "Why," "How," and "What." There are four primary types of qualitative research approaches that are discussed in this chapter—phenomenology, case study, ethnography, and grounded theory (Table 5.5).

Phenomenology aims to understand a phenomenon regarding one's lived experience such as self-perceptions as a medical doctor, diagnostic reasoning ability, experiences of vulnerable populations during medical care, or medical school experience of students from historically marginalized populations. Phenomenological research allows researchers to determine the common human experience.

Case study research examines a case, or a system that is bounded [7]. It "is defined as a systematic investigation that is conducted in a natural setting where the contemporary case or phenomenon has embedded and interacted within its real-life social context, and where the boundary between the case and its context is unclear" (Yin 2014, as cited by ([8], p 1–2).

Ethnographic studies are rooted in the field of anthropology. This type of qualitative research aims to understand the culture of people. For example, an ethnography may aim to understand the patient-physician relationship within an urban free clinic.

Table 5.5 Types of qualitative research

Approach	Example research question	Data collection
Phenomenology	How do Latino/Latina Americans experience medical care in Houston, TX?	Interviews
Case study	Why do medical students at Addis Ababa in Ethiopia plan to emigrate after graduation?	Interviews Focus group Documents
Ethnography	"What are the dynamics of the patient-physician relationship within a New York urban free clinic?	Interviews Participant observation
Grounded theory	What are the experiences of African American males in top-tier US nursing schools?	Interviews Observation Focus groups Documents

In this way, the researcher may use observation and interviews to describe the culture of collaborative care, patient respect, empathy, and/or racial disparities.

Grounded theory research is used for the development or refinement of theory of social phenomena [9] that is rooted (i.e., grounded) in a systematic approach [10]. This process includes methods related to sampling, researcher reflection (i.e., memoing), analysis, and theory building (i.e., theoretical sensitivity).

5.4.1 Sampling

There are three common sampling techniques in qualitative research—convenient, judgmental (purposive), and snowball. Convenience sampling "is the least rigorous technique" of the qualitative sampling approaches ([11], p 523). This approach relies on using anyone who can be easily recruited and available from the population under study. As such, they are selected out of convenience for the researcher. Snowball sampling relies on participants in the study to identify other individuals who might also participate. Just like a snowball that increases in size as it rolls down a snowy mountain, the idea is that the sample size will increase as new participants are recommended by others. Judgmental (purposive sampling) is when the researcher "selects the most productive sample to answer the research question." It is purposeful in that the researcher has known characteristics needed from the population and recruits people from the population with those qualities [1].

5.4.2 Data Collection

Qualitative data includes observation, interviews, focus groups, open-ended survey questions, documents, and images to name a few. This section provides a brief description of the four most common data types for this research paradigm. Further, practices to maximize the quality of each are discussed.

In the medical field, clinical observation is a tool for data gathering that is necessary for learning, documenting, and diagnosing illnesses in patients. In qualitative research, observation is also a tool for data gathering to examine complex interactions, body language, and behaviors. According to Marshall and Rossman [12], observation is the "systematic noting and recording of events, behaviors, and artifacts (objects) in a social setting chosen for study" (p 98). During observation, the researcher collects data using field notes to capture broad areas of interest that align with the research question and purpose.

One type of observation is participant observation. This is used when the researcher is collecting data in a context in which they work or personally interact. Participant observation is the "naturalistic, qualitative research in which the investigator obtains information through relatively intense, prolonged interaction with those being studied and firsthand involvement in the relevant activities of their lives.

The primary data are typically narrative descriptions (i.e., field notes) based on direct observation, informal conversational interviews, and personal experience" ([13], p 38). The two purposes of the participant observer [14] are to engage in activities appropriate to the situation or observe the activities, people, and physical aspects (e.g., faculty meeting, student lounge).

Interviews aim "to understand the world from the subjects' point of view, to unfold the meaning of peoples' experiences, to uncover their lived world …." They allow the researcher to "[l]isten to what people have to say about their lived world, [h]ear people express their opinions in their own words, and [l]earn about the views, dreams, and hopes of others" ([15], p 1). Kvale uses the metaphors of a miner and traveler when describing the interviewer. As a miner, the researcher is trying to unearth valuable information that is buried within the research participant. The knowledge is waiting in the subject's interior to be uncovered, uncontaminated by the miner. The interviewer digs nuggets of data from the experiences of the subject. As a traveler, the researcher is on a journey that leads to a story told at the end of the journey. The traveler wanders through the context, entering into conversations, freely as he/she goes. He/she asks questions as they go, leading subjects to tell the stories of their lived experiences. The researcher aims to construct a story from the journey, which can lead to new knowledge, but it may change the traveler as well leading to new self-awareness, questioning of self, insights, etc. (p 1).

The semi-structured interview is commonly used in social science research. This type of interview has structure and purpose and a strategic approach to questioning and listening. While there are set questions determined by the research prior to the interview, the semi-structured nature of the interview allows for opportunities to ask spontaneous follow-up questions based on the participants' responses to the static questions. Just as with observation, interviewing is systematic. There are common mistakes to avoid when conducting an interview [16]. One is asking closed- instead of open-ended questions. For example, instead of asking "Do you communicate with patients to obtain their medical history?" (closed-ended), ask "How do you communicate with patients to obtain their medical history" (open-ended) or "What is your process for obtaining the medical history of patients?" (open-ended). Another mistake is asking multiple questions at one time. When this is done, the participant may not answer each question completely or respond with the level of depth needed for analysis. Instead, the researcher should ask one question at a time. Another mistake is steering. This is when the researcher overdirects the question, so the participant responds in a way that aligns with the researchers' own ideas, therefore leading to biased findings. To mitigate, the researcher should remain open to all responses to ultimately uncover participants' lived experiences and not their own ideas. The last mistake discussed here is losing track of the interview where the researcher does not remain in control and veers off the path aligned with the research questions and purpose. The researcher must keep these goals (research questions and purpose) at the forefront of the interview. Successful focus groups rely on some of these same skills.

"[F]ocus groups assume that an individual's attitudes and beliefs do not form in a vacuum: People often need to listen to others' opinions and understandings to form their own" ([12], p 114). Focus groups generally include 5–10 participants (ideally 6–8) and include both structured and semi-structured question types. Participants in the focus group often share a common characteristic (e.g., first-year medical students). The nature of a group interview warrants the mention of personality types. It is important that the researcher is aware that the personality types may influence participants' responses during the focus group.

To conduct a successful focus group, the moderator should first create a supportive environment such that participants feel comfortable engaging in the focus group. The researcher/moderator must also be skilled at keeping the conversation on track by managing dominant talkers and personality, shy or introverted respondents, or ramblers. Further, they should avoid value-laden responses that indicate to participants that their answer is "correct." Phrases such as "I agree" or "Excellent" should be avoided.

Open-ended questions on a survey are another way to collect qualitative data. Although this is a quicker approach to collecting perspectives from respondents than interviews or focus groups, they do not allow the researcher to probe deeper. Further, nonresponse is also problematic. However, despite these challenges, there are approaches that may help to collect quality data using open-ended questions on a survey, such as asking open-ended questions, avoiding closed-ended yes/no questions, writing specific questions, sequencing questions so they build upon one another, leaving enough space for in-depth responses, and positioning open-ended questions at the beginning and middle of the questionnaire instead of at the end [17].

5.4.3 Trustworthiness

In qualitative research, the researcher is the research instrument. In other words, they are the medium through which data are filtered. Given this reality, the role of the researcher and the biases they bring to the analysis process are important considerations to minimize. Trustworthiness is an umbrella term for validity and reliability in qualitative research [18], which includes credibility, transferability, dependability, and confirmability. It is important for the researcher to consider each component as they engage in qualitative research.

Credibility is like internal validity in quantitative research. For qualitative studies, credibility signifies the findings aligned with reality. To encourage credibility, approaches such as encouraging honesty/frankness from participants, using research-based data collection approaches for the topic of research, data triangulation (the use of three methods such as interviews, focus groups, and observation), and member checking [19] (a method where participants examine their interviews to ensure accuracy or the analysis to confirm the researchers' interpretation) are useful [20]. Transferability is the transfer of findings to other, but similar contexts. In this way, it is like external validity/generalizability in quantitative research. Dependability in qualitative research is similar to reliability in quantitative research; however, emphasis is given to consistency as it relates to the process instead of the findings [21]. As such, providing a detailed description of the research methods for the sake of replication helps to establish dependability. Finally, confirmability is akin to objectivity in quantitative research. For qualitative research, this means that "steps must be taken to help ensure as far as possible that the work's findings are the result of the experiences and ideas of the informants, rather than the characteristics and preferences of the researcher" [20].

5.4.4 Qualitative Research Analysis

Analysis in qualitative research can take on a variety of forms [22]. The approach taken depends on the type of qualitative research; however, what is common is the iterative nature of data analysis and the ideas of coding and theme development. The iterative process is rooted in the fact that data collection and analysis go hand in hand for the sake of a "coherent interpretation" [12] where the researcher is guided by initial concepts from prior research that can be modified with continued data collection and analysis. Marshall and Rossman offer a seven-step process to qualitative data analysis:

- Step 1: "Organize the Data." Here, the researcher should transcribe the data if needed; perform minor edits to the data; create tables with dates, activity (e.g., focus group, observation, interview, open-ended questionnaire), names, times, places, etc.; and enter the data in a software program.
- Step 2: "Immerse Yourself in the Data." In this step, researchers must read, reread, and read the transcripts, field notes, etc. again. Becoming intimately familiar with the data is necessary for the analysis project.
- Step 3: "Generate Categories and Themes." This is the "process of examining the data for patterns that are evident in the setting (from observation) and expressed by participants (interview, focus groups, open-ended survey questions). The analytic process demands a heightened awareness of the data, a focused attention to those data, and an openness to the subtle, tacit undercurrents of social life. Identifying salient themes, recurring ideas or language, and patterns of belief that link people and settings together is the most intellectually challenging phase of data analysis" ([12], p 159).
- Generating of categories and themes is determined using either emergent intuitive analysis or prefigure technical analysis. The former relies on a loose design where categories are not determined prior to the data analysis. Instead, the researcher relies on their intuitive and interpretive capacities. As such, categories and themes emerge from the data [23]. The researcher may create categories and themes using words expressed by the participants or using words that were not explicitly used by participants, but with meaning grounded in the data. Prefigure technical analysis relies on what is regarded as a tight design such that categories and themes are developed in advance using theory, prior research, and a concep-

tual framework [24]. As such, the researcher relies on "well-delineated constructs and a conceptual framework" (p 19).

- Step 4: "Code the Data." During this step, the researcher applies some coding scheme to the developed categories and themes and diligently and thoroughly marks passages in the data using the codes. A code is a key word or word, colored dot, number, etc. ([12], p 160) that captures the meaning of a segment of the data [1].
- Step 5: "Interpret the Findings." This process requires that the researcher attach "significance to what was found, making sense of the findings, offering explanations, drawing conclusions … and considering meanings …" ([12], p 162). During this step, the researcher also connects the findings to theory [25].
- Step 6: "Search for Alternate Understandings." During this step, the researcher challenges patterns by searching for disconfirming evidence, identifying, and describing alternate explanations (e.g., circumstances when a theme or category does not occur).
- Step 7: "Write the Report." The report for qualitative analysis is a balance between describing the categories, themes, and codes and interpreting the findings. The description often includes vignettes, direct quotes, and tables of themes with examples. Interpreting the findings relies on literature and theory.

5.5 Mixed-Methods Research

Mixed-methods research continues to be a burgeoning area of research [26, 27] and is the third research paradigm discussed in this chapter that brings together the quantitative and qualitative research paradigms. "Mixed-methods research is the type of research in which a researcher or a team of researchers combines elements of qualitative and quantitative research approaches (e.g., use of qualitative and quantitative viewpoints, data collection, analysis, inference techniques) for the broad purposes of breadth and depth of understanding and corroboration" ([28], p 123).

Mixed-methods research is appropriate when one data source is not appropriate or the results from one research paradigm need further exploration using another paradigm. It is inappropriate when the scope of the project is too narrow and does not warrant an additional research paradigm, if the researchers lack an understanding of mixed-methods research, or if it is not feasible to collect quantitative and qualitative data. Further, the research questions and purpose should also warrant the use of mixed-methods research.

Mixed-methods research is used for multiple types of research studies including experimental and nonexperimental studies, case studies, action research, improvement studies, and program evaluation, to name a few. According to Creamer [29], there are six purposes for mixed-methods research:

- Triangulation/confirmation: To enhance validity by using different types of data to measure the same phenomenon (e.g., questionnaire with closed- and open-ended questions).
- Enhancement/complementarity: To gain a deeper and wider understanding for the purposes of generating or testing a theory. This purpose is associated with research questions that ask what, how, and/or why (e.g., merging qualitative and quantitative data in one dataset).
- Development: To develop an instrument, enhance participant selection, and get information to customize an intervention to a setting (e.g., observations or interview data followed by the development and pilot testing of an instrument).
- Initiation: To examine extreme or negative cases or explore unexpected or contradictory findings (e.g., testing competing hypotheses).
- Multilevel/expansion: To study multilevel systems such as a medical system or to examine nested designs or make cross-case comparisons (e.g., students within classrooms, medical schools within states, faculty within medical schools).
- Evaluation/intervention/process oriented: To examine the effectiveness of an intervention and provide contextual understanding (e.g., collect participant data to design an intervention for a particular context, collect data to examine the effectiveness of the intervention and provide contextual understanding).

5.5.1 Fully Integrated and Quasi-Mixed-Methods Studies

The general and specific research purpose and subsequent research questions are addressed in mixed-methods research using either a fully integrated mixed-methods study or a quasi-mixed study [29]. The degree of integration is determined by the level of mixing across the phases of research (i.e., research purpose, research questions, data collection, data analysis, and drawing conclusions) (Table 5.6). According to Creamer (p 6), "*[m]ixing is the linking, merging, or embedding of qualitative and quantitative strands of a mixed methods study.* It is not present when the strands [qualitative and quantitative] of a mixed study are kept parallel or distinct." A fully integrated study mixes the quantitative and qualitative strands across all phases of research. The strands are kept separate for a quasi-mixed methods study. In this case, multiple data sources answer different questions, and these sources are not mixed within the research phases.

5.5.2 Timing and Priority

Given that both quantitative and qualitative data are collected, priority and timing are essential elements of mixed-methods research. Studies can have quantitative dominant status, qualitative dominant status, or equal status. The notation identifies the dominant research paradigm, which is written in all caps (e.g., QUAN, QUAL),

Table 5.6 Fully integrated mixed-methods study

Research phase	Description
Research purpose	Articulates the "what" and "why" of the phenomenon of interest
Research questions	A question, aligned to the research purpose that aims to examine: *Blending into a single statement*[a] e.g.: What are the implications of MCAT preparation courses on medical school acceptance? *Separate but linked research questions* e.g.: (1) How do medical school faculty respond to the flipped classroom approach to learning? (2) To what extent is the faculty response associated with student outcomes? *An explicitly labeled mixing question* e.g.: (Mixed) Do the values endorsed in mission statements (qualitatively derived) differ between institutions with lower and higher than average enrollment of women (quantitatively derived)?
Data collection	"Mixed-method sampling procedures use various approaches to combine a traditional quantitative (i.e., probability) approach to sampling with a qualitative (i.e., purposeful) approach"[b] *Concurrent mixed-methods sampling* • Single sample of participants • Qualitative and quantitative data collected simultaneously and around the same time point *Sequential mixed-methods sampling* • Subsequent sampling strategy is directly linked to the results of analytical procedures earlier in the study
Data analysis	Mixing both data types to identify, compare, and consolidate similar findings around common themes.[b] There are four types of analysis: • Blending • Converting • Cross-case comparison • Meta-inferences
Drawing conclusions	The process of data interpretation through the connection to the literature

[a][30, 31]
[b][29], p 89

while the paradigm with less priority is written in lower case letters (e.g., quan, qual). In addition to priority, the timing of the quantitative and qualitative paradigms is an important consideration. Qualitative and quantitative data can be collected concurrently (denoted by +) or sequentially (denoted by →). For example, a QUAN + qual mixed-methods study is quantitative dominant and the quantitative and qualitative data are collected concurrently. A QUAL → quan study is qualitative dominant where the quantitative data is collected after the qualitative data has been collected and analyzed.

5.5.3 Designs

There are several design typologies for mixed-methods research. One popular typology was developed by Creswell and Plano Clark [2]. Their typology includes three core designs—the convergent, explanatory, and exploratory designs.

The convergent design uses complementary data. In this way, the strengths of both quantitative and qualitative methods are utilized such that overlapping weaknesses are minimized. As a result, comparisons and validations can be made between statistical results and qualitative findings. The convergent design is a one-phase (concurrent), equal-weight approach. Quantitative and qualitative methods are collected at the same time, and both methods receive equal weight throughout the process for a shared purpose [32]. Taken together (timing and paradigm dominance), the convergent design uses a QUAL + QUAN approach.

The strengths of this design lie in the efficiency of the one-phase approach and the potential independence of each paradigm during analysis. One challenge is the required level of knowledge, and pragmatic application is an attribute that research purists often do not possess. Further analyzing data sample sizes that may vary tremendously may also challenge the researcher. Finally, another challenge of this design is the fact that researchers must resolve conflicting results between both data types [2].

The explanatory design is a two-phase (sequential) quantitative dominant design—QUAN → qual [2]. This design is used primarily when researchers want to explain significant or nonsignificant quantitative results, outliers, or unanticipated results using qualitative research. Therefore, phase one requires the collection and analysis of quantitative data, while the second qualitative phase connects to the quantitative findings.

The strength of this design is rooted in a straightforward implementation due to the two-phase approach in which the two methods of data collection occur in separate phases [33]. The weaknesses of this design stem from the required time necessary to collect and analyze data across two phases, sampling decisions and difficulties with the internal review board. The inability to specify the selection of participants for phase two without the results from phase one grounds the latter weakness for the explanatory design (p 75).

The exploratory design is similar to the explanatory design because of its two-phase approach. However, the exploratory design is most commonly qualitative dominant- QUAL → quan. Here, a phenomenon must be explored prior to quantitative exploration. This design is appropriate when instruments are unavailable, variables cannot be specified, or when a framework or theory does not exist [33]. Variants of this design reflect differences in the dominance of the qualitative paradigm during data collection and final analysis. For example, designs used for instrument development may utilize a qual → QUAN design. Qualitative data is collected first, but to support the quantitative dominant study.

5.5.4 Mixed-Methods Research Analysis

The goal of analyzing mixed-methods data is to identify, compare, and consolidate similar result findings around common themes [29]. There are several approaches to analyzing data for mixed-methods research. Creamer describes four general approaches—blending, converting, cross-case analysis, and meta-inferences.

Blending is an approach where a variable, category, or theme is generated from one type of analysis and tested with a different data type. In a different instance, a variable, category, or factor is created by combining qualitative and quantitative data.

Converting is a strategy where data is transformed. Here, the researchers use data consolidation where qualitative and data are converted to quantitative data or vice versa. For this, we use an example of a study that aimed to examine faculty's perceptions of the flipped classroom (qualitative) and how their perceptions influenced students' self-directed learning [34] (quantitative). Veering some from the actual study findings, if the qualitative findings revealed that the perceptions were captured by themes of enhancement and reduction in self-regulated learning, then one might take that qualitative data and convert it to a nominal variable. In this way, faculty with the perception of enhancement are given a 1 and faculty with the perception of reduction are given a 2. This allows for quantitative comparisons in students' self-directed learning scores. The researcher is able to examine differences in self-regulated learning between the two faculty perceptions. This is called quantitizing.

Qualitizing is when for example measures on a quantitative instrument are summarized in narrative form. For example, when a researcher uses the qualitative data to summarize what each Likert item entails for self-regulated learning (e.g., not at all, somewhat, most of the time), they are qualitizing quantitative data. For example, when asked about the flipped classroom, the researcher could qualitize the quantitative data to show what somewhat or most of the time entails.

Another way to analyze the data is through cross-case comparisons where qualitative and quantitative data are consolidated by creating profiles. This approach is used to test or extend upon qualitatively or quantitatively derived themes for the purpose of comparison. For example, a researcher may examine a medical school in which faculty readily use the flipped classroom as an instructional approach and one medical school where the traditional lecture is the norm. Here, the researcher might compare the two schools and create profiles using quantitative and qualitative data.

Meta-inference links, compares, and contrasts quantitative and qualitative findings. A meta-inference is a conclusion generated by integrating inferences from the qual and quan strand of a study. It links the findings from qual and quan in an explanatory way. In the end, the researcher is able to make an assertation that explains the connection between the two data types.

5.6 Conclusion

Research questions and purposes are addressed using quantitative, qualitative, and mixed-methods research in varying ways. While each research paradigm has strengths and weaknesses, they are rooted in rigorous methods. This chapter provides insight on the approaches that will help the novice researcher choose appropriate methods that will minimize bias within the research study.

5.7 Questions

Discussion Questions
1. Classify the following as discrete or continuous variables:

   (a) Blood pressure
   (b) Patients presenting with uncontrolled hypertension to a medical practice within a 6-month period
   (c) Student exam scores
   (d) Quality in healthcare

Activities
1. Identify variables relevant to your research project.
2. Using the research question you have developed so far, choose a research paradigm and state why it is appropriate.

   (Discussion Question Answers: Continuous, Discrete, Discrete, Continuous)

References

1. Johnson B, Christensen LB. Educational research: quantitative, qualitative, and mixed approaches. Thousand Oaks: Sage; 2014.
2. Creswell JW, Plano Clark VL. Designing and conducting mixed methods research. Thousand Oaks: Sage; 2018.
3. Nagel T. The view from nowhere. Oxford: Oxford University Press; 1989.
4. Johnson RB, Onwuegbuzie AJ. Mixed methods research: a research paradigm whose time has come. Educ Res. 2004;33(7):14–26. https://doi.org/10.3102/0013189x033007014.
5. Michael K, Dror MG, Karnieli-Miller O. Students' patient-centered-care attitudes: the contribution of self-efficacy, communication, and empathy. Patient Educ Couns. 2019;102(11):2031–7. https://doi.org/10.1016/j.pec.2019.06.004.
6. Shadish WR, Cook TD, Campbell DT. Experimental and quasi-experimental designs for generalized causal inference. Boston: Wadsworth Cengage Learning; 2002.
7. Stake RE. The art of case study research. Thousand Oaks: Sage; 1995.
8. Nilmanat K, Kurniawan T. The quest in case study research. Pac Rim Int J Nurs. 2019;25(1):1–6.
9. Glaser BG, Strauss A. The discovery of grounded theory: strategies for qualitative research. Aldine Publishing Co.; 1967.

10. Chun Tie Y, Birks M, Francis K. Grounded theory research: a design framework for novice researchers. SAGE Open Med. 2019;7:205031211882292. https://doi.org/10.1177/2050312118822927.

11. Marshall MN. Sampling for qualitative research. Fam Pract. 1996;13(6):522–5.

12. Marshall C, Rossman GB. Designing qualitative research. Thousand Oaks: Sage; 2006.

13. Levine HG, Gallimore R, Weisner TS, Turner JL. Teaching participant-observation research methods: a skills-building approach. Anthropol Educ Q. 1980;11(1):38–54. https://doi.org/10.1525/aeq.1980.11.1.05x1849c.

14. Spradley JP. The ethnographic interview. Holt, Rinehart, and Winston; 1979.

15. Kvale S. Interviews: an introduction to qualitive research interviewing. Sage; 1996.

16. Gesch-Karamanlidis E. Reflecting on novice qualitative interviewer mistakes. The Qualitative Report. 2015. https://doi.org/10.46743/2160-3715/2015.2145.

17. Galesic M, Bosnjak M. Effects of questionnaire length on participation and indicators of response quality in a web survey. Public Opin Q. 2009;73(2):349–60. https://doi.org/10.1093/poq/nfp031.

18. Guba EG. Criteria for assessing the trustworthiness of naturalistic inquiries. ECTJ. 1981;29(2). https://doi.org/10.1007/bf02766777.

19. Birt L, Scott S, Cavers D, Campbell C, Walter F. Member checking. *Qualitative Health Research*. 2016;26(13):1802–1811. https://doi.org/10.1177/1049732316654870.

20. Shenton AK. Strategies for ensuring trustworthiness in qualitative research projects. Educ Inf. 2004;22(2):63–75. https://doi.org/10.3233/efi-2004-22201.

21. Lincoln YS, Guba EG. Naturalistic inquiry. Sage; 1985.

22. Coffey A, Atkinson P. Making sense of qualitative data: complementary research strategies. Sage; 1996.

23. Erickson F. Qualitative methods in research on teaching. In: Wittrock MC, editor. Handbook of research on teaching. Macmillan; 1986. p. 119–59.

24. Miles MB, Huberman AM, Saldaña J. Qualitative data analysis: a methods sourcebook. Sage; 2014.

25. Wolcott HF. Writing up qualitative research. Sage; 2001.

26. Bergman MM. Advances in mixed methods research: theories and applications. Thousand Oaks: Sage; 2008.

27. Leech NL, Onwuegbuzie AJ. A typology of mixed methods research designs. Qual Quantity Int J Methodol. 2009;43(2):265–75. https://doi.org/10.1007/s11135-007-9105-3.

28. Johnson RB, Onwuegbuzie AJ, Turner LA. Toward a definition of mixed methods research. J Mixed Methods Res. 2007;1(2):112–33. https://doi.org/10.1177/1558689806298224.

29. Creamer EG. An introduction to fully integrated mixed methods research. Thousand Oaks: Sage; 2018.

30. Plano Clark VL, Badiee M. Research questions in mixed methods research. In: Tashakkori A, Teddlie C, editors. Handbook of mixed methods research. 2nd ed. Thousand Oaks: Sage; 2010.

31. Onwuegbuzie A, Leech N. Linking research questions to mixed methods data analysis procedures. Qual Rep. 2006;11(3):474–98. https://doi.org/10.46743/2160-3715/2006.1663.

32. Ridenour CS, Newman I. Mixed methods research: exploring the interactive continuum. Carbondale: Southern Illinois University Press; 2008.

33. Creswell JW, Plano Clark VL. Designing and conducting mixed methods research. Thousand Oaks: Sage; 2007.

34. Ramnanan C, Pound L. Advances in medical education and practice: student perceptions of the flipped classroom. Adv Med Educ Pract. 2017;8:63–73. https://doi.org/10.2147/amep.s109037.

Part III
Examining Impact

Chapter 6
Evaluation Paradigms

Serkan Toy

6.1 Introduction

Evaluation is a key component of educational scholarship endeavors including, but not limited to, curriculum development, program evaluation, and educational research. Similar to the decisions we make in research, what and how we evaluate largely depend on our theoretical assumptions and value judgments. In his influential book *"The Structure of Scientific Revolutions,"* Kuhn describes the paradigm as *"the entire constellation of beliefs, values, techniques, and so on shared by the members of a given community"* ([1], p 175).

There are several paradigms that guide research and evaluation efforts in health professions education. In this book, the focus is on the practical applications of evaluation in the context of educational scholarship. Herein, paradigms are conceptual frameworks that guide evaluation efforts logically and systematically. Some of the evaluation frameworks discussed in this chapter include Bloom's taxonomy [2], Miller's pyramid [3], Kirkpatrick's four-step model [4], and evaluation component of the six-step approach to curriculum development [5]. More detailed philosophical and theoretical accounts surrounding ontological, epistemological, and axiological perspectives are beyond the scope of this chapter but available in a series titled the "Philosophy of Science" in Academic Medicine journal (see Varpio and MacLeod [6]).

S. Toy (✉)
Departments of Basic Science Education & Health Systems and Implementation Science, Virginia Tech Carilion School of Medicine, Roanoke, VA, USA
e-mail: serkantoy@vt.edu

A. S. Fitzgerald, G. Bosch (eds.), *Education Scholarship in Healthcare*,
https://doi.org/10.1007/978-3-031-38534-6_6

6.2 Terminology and Concepts

There are several concepts and terminology related to evaluation. *Evaluation for scholarship* differs from *curricular* or *program evaluation* mainly by its intended audience. While curricular or program evaluation is performed specifically to improve the curriculum and to inform the stakeholders, in the case of evaluation for scholarship, the audience goes beyond those immediate stakeholders. To contribute to the knowledge base on a given topic, you need to take the additional step of disseminating your findings.

Evaluation is sometimes used interchangeably with *assessment* or *measurement*, but they are different. An assessment or measurement is an act of quantifying or assigning a numerical index to an individual's knowledge, skills, or attitude; it is about the individual learner. Evaluation determines the extent to which an educational intervention has met its goal and objectives, often by using measurements such as learner assessments—questionnaires, knowledge tests, checklists, rubrics, and the like.

Evaluation efforts are often classified under two main categories depending on the intended use. *Formative evaluation* is typically carried out to improve the educational intervention, and *summative evaluation* is used to determine whether a given modality should be offered again. In the context of a scholarly project, evaluation could serve both purposes depending on the project goals.

Assessment or measurement can be based either on external criteria (*criterion-referenced*) or in relation to other individuals (*norm-referenced*). Most often, measurement in the context of health professions education is criterion-referenced using clearly defined criteria such as a competency-based framework.

You will often hear about *psychometrics* in the context of educational measurement. Most variables (or constructs) in educational and psychological research cannot be measured directly. We often operationalize rather abstract constructs into variables by quantifying knowledge, skills, or attitudes based on responses to psychological measures (e.g., knowledge tests, checklists, or questionnaires). Psychometrics is an applied field of study that deals with the systematic development and validation of measurement tools providing rigor and credibility for evaluation results. *Reliability* and *validity* are two main concepts that help with quality assurance for measurement. Reliability provides information regarding the extent to which a tool is consistently measuring across time and observers, while validity refers to whether the tool actually measures the construct that it intends to measure. These concepts will be further discussed later in this chapter.

Additionally, several terms are used interchangeably in this chapter. These are *assessment tool*, *instrument*, and *measure*. They typically refer to a specific questionnaire, a multiple-choice knowledge test, or an observational checklist. Sometimes, *survey* and *questionnaire* can be used synonymously; however, questionnaire is used in this chapter to indicate an assessment tool since survey can mean an entire research methodology beyond a specific instrument. Although there is some nuance, *scale*, *inventory*, and *questionnaire* are often used interchangeably.

6.3 Where to Begin?

The research question and outcomes of interest will drive the evaluation efforts for the scholarly project. Evaluation does not start after the teaching and learning activities have finished. Instead, evaluation begins when we start developing the research questions and learning outcomes. Outcomes guide the evaluation plan. Once a good scholarship question has been identified, Bloom's taxonomy [7] and Miller's pyramid can provide guidance while formulating the outcomes for the educational intervention [3]. See Fig. 6.1.

These frameworks are useful for aligning intervention objectives and assessment tools. At the base of the Miller's pyramid are knowledge categories related to factual and applied clinical knowledge (knows and knows how, respectively), whereas the top two relate to demonstration of skills during an observed assessment situation and a judgment of competency to practice independently in real-life clinical settings (shows how and does, respectively). Moreover, Bloom's taxonomy further helps detail different aspects of cognitive skills moving from lower order to higher order cognitive skills. This taxonomy could make it easier to align assessment tools with the intended learning outcomes and thus evaluate the effectiveness of the intervention.

In the remainder of this chapter, the activities for the evaluation component of a scholarly project are discussed. While there may be some logical sequence to their completion, these efforts inform one another, necessitating some iteration, especially during the discovery/planning phase. For example, sample size considerations may inform the researcher to re-examine the target learner population or, while

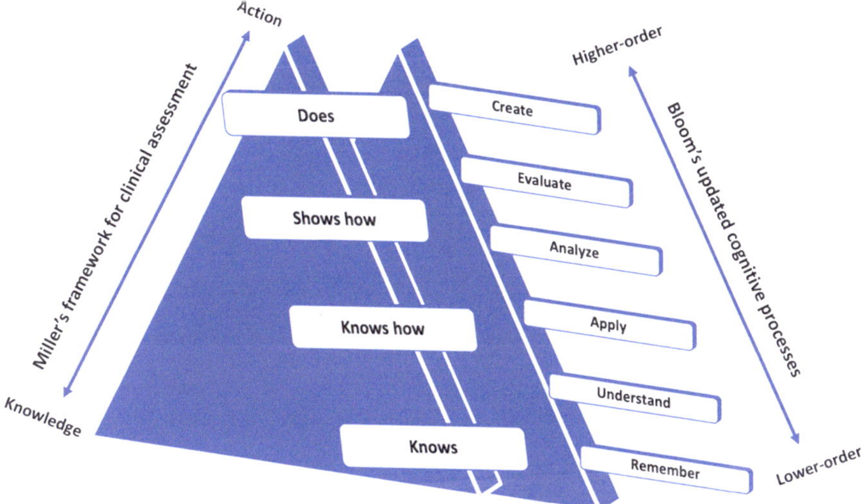

Fig. 6.1 Miller's framework for clinical assessment alongside of Bloom's taxonomy of the cognitive processes

identifying specific measures, outcomes can be revisited and finetuned. See Table 6.1 for a quick guide to evaluation activities.

6.4 Discovery/Planning Phase

Many projects begin with an observation of a performance gap in a group of health-related learners, e.g., patients, trainees, faculty, or staff. This performance gap prompts educators to identify an educational intervention they would like to make. The first step is to understand the target learner population.

Table 6.1 Quick guide for evaluation activities

1. Discovery phase/evaluation plan
   - Examine target population
   - Determine evaluation design (similar to research design)
   - Identify and compile measures (Kirkpatrick model can be helpful; published instruments, any objective measures—sensors from simulators, etc.)
   - Consider statistical techniques/analyses (sample size/power calculations, statistical tests)
   - Consider ethical issues (cannot deny education, high monetary incentives, evaluator in an authority role, any potential for coercion or undue influence or selection/response bias)
2. Action (developing and pilot testing measures and collecting data)
   - Develop needed measures (questionnaires, checklists, rubrics, knowledge tests, or interview or focus group protocols, coding schemes, etc.)
     - Literature search
     - Delphi technique
   - Pilot test instruments
     - Examine reliability and validity
     - Examine knowledge test difficulty and discrimination
     - Questionnaire—clear and concise (cognitive interview)
     - Train and calibrate raters
   - *Reflection in action (here one can make the final revisions and get ready for prime time)*
   - Data collection (response methods, response rate, reminders)
3. Analysis
   - Examine data quality, missing data, and outliers
   - Determine how to handle missing data (despite best evaluation design, intentions, and efforts, one will face the challenges of dealing with missing or incomplete data in educational evaluation)
   - Develop tables and/or figures for descriptive data (demographics, responses to Likert-scale items)
   - Examine assumptions for parametric tests
   - Run statistical tests
4. Reflection on action: reporting evaluation results
This is where you reflect back on all evaluation efforts and results and synthesize them relative to the rest of the scholarly project

6.4.1 Examination of the Target Learner Population

A needs assessment of the targeted learners guides the educational intervention and outcomes of the scholarship project, and this information will help determine how an intervention should be evaluated [8]. A needs assessment involves finding out details of what the target learner population already knows and what still can be improved on in their knowledge, skills, and attitudes to address the identified educational need. During this process, evaluators can also determine to what extent the educational intervention is likely to make a difference in the targeted outcomes. While an intended educational intervention could address an educational gap, there might not be a change in the related outcomes. This could be caused by the intervention not being effective, caused by factors outside of the intervention, or partially by both the intervention not being fully effective and outside factors. Thus, exploring barriers and ways to mitigate those can be critical at this stage.

6.4.2 Evaluation Design

We now focus on determining an effective and feasible data collection scheme for a robust and compelling evaluation. This section is intended to provide a brief and practical guide to introduce the main evaluation design schemes that can be used in health professions education. In educational research, many different variations of the designs discussed below exist, which could inform evaluation design as well.

The crucial aspect of evaluation design is to strike a balance between what is essential to evaluate and what is feasible. All essential elements of the scholarly project (outcomes) should be evaluated without redundancy. Aligning outcomes, data collection schemes, and measurement tools will help save time and energy during the analysis and reporting phases. It is always intriguing to collect more data, but often redundant data will cause noise and make it challenging to identify pertinent trends and focus on the key findings. Therefore, any data that does not relate to the given scholarly questions should probably be excluded.

Scholarship projects in health professions education are typically embedded in real-life settings. This can be a strength for evaluation as the results can provide practical implications for clinical educators (external validity). However, real-life environments are often replete with many factors that are not considered and measured as part of the scholarship project. Conducting evaluation in a real-life setting limits the ability to control these potentially confounding factors and introduces a number of threats that could weaken the evaluation design (internal validity). Similar to educational research studies, history, maturation, measurement exposure, instrumentation, selection, dropout, and intervention diffusion could pose some threats to the evaluation design.

6.4.2.1 Threats to Evaluation Design

History This can be an issue, especially when pretest, intervention(s), and post-measurements are spread across several weeks to months. There is a chance that learners may get exposed to the key knowledge and skills related to the intervention during other educational lectures, teaching rounds, or clinical service. This could confound the evaluation results. It is a good practice to ask participants to list related experience or learning that occurred between the pretest and posttest but was outside the intervention. This practice can partially address the issue. Additionally, having a control group that may have been exposed to similar learning conditions could alleviate this threat.

Maturation In the context of health professions education, maturation can be similar to history. However, maturation refers specifically to the changes that take place within the participants during the course of the study as opposed to exposure to other specific educational offerings. For example, first-year anesthesiology residents may feel more confident to speak up with a patient management concern during surgeries towards the end of the year compared to earlier in the year. In part, this may be due to residents becoming more comfortable in their role and finding their voice within the health care team. However, scheduled lectures and clinical learning experiences could play a role in this as well (history). Similar to history, including a control group could control for maturation.

Measurement Exposure (Testing) If the same assessment tool such as a knowledge test or a simulation scenario is used multiple times (e.g., pretest and posttest), the posttest results could be different simply due to this exposure.

Instrumentation Sometimes, different assessment tools are used at the pretest and posttest to prevent participants from getting familiar with the assessment tool. However, the difficulty level and the actual content of the tools (a knowledge test or a simulation scenario) may not be exactly the same. This makes the interpretation of evaluation results problematic as the observed variability between the pretest and posttest could be due to the change in the assessment tools.

Selection Imbalanced distribution of participants by gender, age, prior experience, etc. within different learning conditions (e.g., control and intervention) could influence the evaluation results beyond the actual intervention effect. Stratified randomization could help address this concern where participants are stratified into subgroups with known similar characteristics and then simply randomized into experimental groups with a balanced representation.

Dropout (Mortality) Sometimes, participants complete pretest measures but do not return for the posttest measurements. This is quite normal for an evaluation conducted in the health professions education as participants are often busy clinicians. However, it becomes an issue when participants who drop out are systematically different than those who complete all measures and/or if they differentially drop out of the control and intervention groups. It is a good practice to investigate if there may be an underlying issue related to intervention, control, or measurement in the event that there is a high dropout rate.

Intervention Diffusion It is possible that participants in the control group work closely with those in the intervention group and may learn certain aspects of the intervention simply by observing their peers or colleagues and adopting similar techniques in their practice. This could be an issue especially if the evaluation takes place over a period of time.

6.4.2.2 Evaluation Design Considerations

There are a number of different design schemes that can be used for data collection to evaluate an educational scholarship project. These have different features making some of them more and some less appropriate or feasible for certain scholarly projects. Overall, the following features are important to consider while deciding on a specific evaluation design.

Baseline Measurement To evaluate the effectiveness of an intervention, we need to measure learners' current level of knowledge, skills, and attitudes before the intervention. This allows for a frame of reference to compare against measures collected post-intervention. Sometimes, when health professions learners complete evaluation-related activities, they may also get exposed to the intended content, and thus it could be considered a part of the intervention as well. For example, a simulation-based assessment of team skills during a code could potentially expose learners to key knowledge and skills and reveal the project objective. Sometimes, evaluators may want to avoid such situations and use a posttest-only design.

Control Group When evaluation results show learning gain, this could be associated with several other factors mentioned above (history, maturation, etc.) besides the educational intervention. Including a control group can isolate the intervention effect in reference to the comparison group. While it is common practice to have a placebo group in clinical research, good practice in educational evaluation is to provide an alternative educational offering (standard education) for the comparison group.

Randomization Randomizing learners into educational conditions is critical as it helps to control for external factors, ensure that groups are comparable, and minimize bias.

The following symbols will be used while illustrating different evaluation designs:

I:	Intervention
IG:	Intervention group
CG:	Control group
M:	Measurement
R:	Randomization

1. *Single group designs*

(a) One-shot case study (single measurement): This design is one of the least desired data collection schemes as it does not provide strong evidence for the evaluation results. The reason why it is called a case study is because it looks like a clinical case study where a measurement of an outcome follows an intervention. This data collection scheme should be avoided if the ultimate goal is to publish the evaluation results indicating the efficacy of an intervention. There may be several external factors confounding the results in this design (e.g., history, maturation, selection, dropout). However, this may be a good way to conduct a pilot test for examining the measurement tools and fine-tuning intervention. This design looks like the following:

I	M_{post}	

(b) Pretest-posttest design: This scheme provides an opportunity to measure a difference in the outcome before and after the intervention by adding a pretest. One argument may be that the participants are serving as their own control. This may work if the time between the pretest and posttest is not long (against history and maturation) and the same assessment tools are being used (against instrumentation). However, this is still susceptible to multiple measurement exposure, and not having a true control group weakens the evidence quality. It is challenging to make a compelling case that the observed evaluation results are associated with the intervention and not partially caused by the confounders due to the inability to isolate the intervention effect in reference to a comparison group. This data collection scheme looks like the following:

M_{pre}	I	M_{post}

(c) Longitudinal repeated measures design—time series design: Most research textbooks will call this type of design a time series design or interrupted time series. This data collection scheme requires multiple measurements and sophisticated analysis (i.e., time-series analysis). However, it can identify different patterns in the outcome of interest over time and create prediction models. In some instances, this design could be useful to examine temporal changes in clinical skills (or competency development). This data scheme might look like the following:

M_1	M_2	M_3	…	M_{15}	I	M_{16}	M_{17}	M_{18}	…	M_{30}

2. *Non-randomized control group design (in other words, quasi-experimental or nonequivalent)*

In health professions education, it is not always possible to randomly assign individuals to different learning conditions. Although having a control group controls for history, maturation, and measurement exposure, randomization would still be needed to control for selection bias. This design can have several different variations. The two most common ones are the pretest-posttest control group and the posttest-only control group.

CG:	M_{pre}		M_{post}
IG:	M_{pre}	I	M_{post}

Sometimes, there can be more than one intervention being evaluated using this scheme, which could be shown as below:

or

CG:	M_{pre}		M_{post}
IG$_1$:	M_{pre}	I_1	M_{post}
IG$_2$:	M_{pre}	I_2	M_{post}

or

IG$_1$:	M_{pre}	I_1	M_{post}
IG$_2$:	M_{pre}	I_2	M_{post}
IG$_3$:	M_{pre}	I_3	M_{post}

3. *Randomized control group design*

Similar to non-randomized designs, this can have several different variations as well. The two most common ones are the pretest-posttest randomized control group and the posttest-only randomized control group.

R	CG:	M_{pre}		M_{post}
	IG:	M_{pre}	I	M_{post}

or

R	CG:		M_{post}
	IG:	I	M_{post}

Sometimes, there can be more than one intervention being evaluated and in a randomized control group design, which could be shown as below:

R	CG:	M_{pre}		M_{post}
	IG_1:	M_{pre}	I_1	M_{post}
	IG_2:	M_{pre}	I_2	M_{post}

In educational settings, there is an obligation to provide educational benefits to all learners, and sometimes randomized control group evaluation design could limit the ability to offer the same education to all learners. Thus, occasionally, evaluators use a crossover design in a randomized control design to provide the benefits of the intervention to the control group. This data collection could be represented as follows:

R	CG:	M_{pre}		M_{post}	I
	IG:	M_{pre}	I	M_{post}	

4. Time series: longitudinal repeated measures randomized control group design

This scheme adds a randomized control group to the single-group time series design discussed previously.

R	CG	M_1	M_2	M_3		M_4	M_5	M_6
	IG	M_1	M_2	M_3	I	M_4	M_5	M_6

6.4.3 Identify and Compile Measures

As discussed previously, aligning objectives/outcomes, intervention, evaluation design, and measures is an effective and efficient way to conduct an educational scholarship project. What types of assessment tools are needed can be determined based on the intended outcomes. Below is a discussion of assessment instruments based on three broad categories: knowledge, skills, and attitudes.

Measuring Knowledge (Cognitive Skills) Written exams are typically used to measure knowledge in a given topic. These exams could be tests with multiple-choice questions (MCQs) or written essays. MCQ tests are typically useful for lower level cognitive skills (e.g., recall and comprehension), and written essays can tap into higher order skills (application, analysis, etc.). It is critical to ensure that the test includes a balanced number of items addressing different levels of cognitive skills. This could provide an opportunity to examine whether and to what extent a knowledge gap exists across the continuum. Performance on factual questions lacks clinical context and may not provide useful information regarding the learners' ability to apply their knowledge in a clinical environment.

- *Multiple-choice questions* (MCQs) can be used as objective measures of knowledge and usually are the easiest to administer and score as there is no rater bias involved. It is also easy to measure learners' breadth of knowledge using a single test with several MCQs on each pertinent concept in a broad range of topics. MCQs can be purely factual and only require recall and understanding. However, some questions can be context rich (using clinical vignettes) and could require the application of medical knowledge or even sometimes analysis and evaluation of a given clinical case. While it is easier to write MCQs measuring facts, it is much harder to write high-quality test questions tapping into higher order cognitive skills. Knowledge tests used for evaluation purposes should go through rigorous development and pilot testing. At a minimum, the test should have an acceptable level of internal consistency, and the test items (MCQs) should show an appropriate level of difficulty and discrimination indices for the target population. It is a good idea to identify previously published standardized tests that can be used for evaluating a given scholarship project. However, it will still be necessary to examine previously published tests' internal consistency, difficulty, and discrimination indices to ensure that they are appropriate for measuring the intended cognitive skills for a given project and target population. It is also critical to provide some validity evidence that the test is actually measuring the intended topic. More discussion on validity evidence will be provided later in the chapter.
- *Essay-type written exams* are used much less frequently compared to MCQs. These questions can provide a brief description of a clinical case and ask the learners to apply their medical knowledge to evaluating and deciding on a treatment plan with rationale (higher order cognitive skills: application, analysis, and evaluation). These exams take more time to administer, and scoring is not as objective as MCQs due to some potential rater bias. Examining and demonstrating an acceptable level of interrater reliability are critical for this type of measurement. It is a good practice to use a well-developed rubric with descriptors for each score level to increase interrater reliability.
- *Oral exams* can also be used to measure more clinically relevant higher order cognitive skills. Some licensing and certification boards in the United States and around the world use high-stakes standardized oral exams for making licensing or certification decisions. These tests have consequences for medical practice and thus require a considerable amount of resources for development and administration as well as highly compelling reliability and validity evidence. However, evaluation for a scholarship project is not typically such a high-stakes enterprise and can use similar methods to measure clinical knowledge with less burden of proof. These exams can take several different formats, for example, oral case presentations or chart-stimulated recall where trainees are asked to provide differential diagnoses and clinical management strategies for a given case. Similar

to written essay-type exams, these require the use of rubrics and multiple raters to establish interrater reliability.

Measuring Skills (Technical/Procedural and Interpersonal Communication Skills) Clinical skills are best observed during patient encounters. These skills include technical/procedural skills as well as team and communication skills. Most institutions collect information from supervising clinicians regarding observed learner patient care skills. However, challenges in this data include inconsistent/infrequent observations as well as diversity in the complexity of these clinical encounters. Additionally, supervising clinicians represent diverse perspectives, and their observations might lack standardization which could render such data less than optimal for evaluating a scholarship project. Standardized patients and/or simulation-based assessments are an alternative for measuring clinical skills. Such settings reduce the complexity and unpredictability inherent in an actual clinical setting.

- *Technical skills:* Skills such as endotracheal intubation and arterial line placement can be observed during simulated exercises and assessed using analytical checklists that include the pertinent steps of the targeted procedures. Sometimes, a global rating scale is used instead of a checklist, but it may be better to use both in combination as they may produce complementary information (a checklist focuses on each critical action, and global scale looks at the overall performance). In recent years, virtual reality, augmented reality, and mixed-reality simulations have become popular for training and assessing technical skills. Some of these simulators include sensors that provide objective metrics as actionable feedback for improvement and can be used for measurement purposes.
- *Team and communication skills:* Communication skills and especially team skills can be challenging to measure effectively. These require well-developed, standardized scenarios and robust checklists and/or rubrics as well as trained raters for producing high-quality data for evaluation purposes. For team skills, the unit of analysis is typically the whole team, and sometimes providing sufficient power for this type of project can be challenging.
- *Objective structured clinical examinations (OSCEs)*: OSCEs are used for medical licensing exams in some countries and can be useful for measuring a range of knowledge and skills as well. These exams may take a considerable amount of time and resources to develop and administer but can be an effective way to measure multiple different levels of medical knowledge, technical skills, and communication skills.

Attitude Sometimes, one of the objectives of the educational intervention is to improve competency beliefs or attitudes towards an issue related to health care. As discussed previously, this type of evidence is the weakest for evaluating a scholarship project. Typically, questionnaires are used for measuring attitudes. It is critical to conduct a literature search and identify relevant previously published questionnaires. A single questionnaire may not measure all aspects of targeted attitudes or perceptions for a given project. Thus, a few scales are often used in combination. If the original scales are used, providing internal consistency evidence (i.e., Cronbach's alpha) could be sufficient, but revising a questionnaire in some way may require a re-examination of the factor structure.

Effectiveness Kirkpatrick's four-step model provides a useful framework for evaluating the effectiveness of an educational scholarship project. This framework examines a given educational intervention at four main levels—reaction, knowledge, behavior, and results. Reaction is related to learner satisfaction and is often measured by a posttest questionnaire. The second level examines the improvement in the knowledge, skills, and attitudes due to the intervention. As discussed previously, learning can be measured in many different ways depending on the outcomes. The third level, behavior, examines to what extent learning gain has actually been transferred into the workplace environment. Direct observations can be used to measure behavior; however, in certain situations, interviews, focus groups, or even self-report questionnaires could be used to examine how often learners had a chance to put their learning to use. The fourth level and hardest to measure is results associated with the intervention. This is similar to asking whether simulation-based training on difficult airways resulted in better patient outcomes. Table 6.2 shows how outcomes, intervention, and assessment align across all four steps of the framework.

Once measures are aligned with the outcomes of interest, the next comes the decision of what specific instruments to use. When no previously published assessment tools can be found addressing the outcomes of a given project, you might need to develop one. Considerations for constructing assessment tools are discussed in the next Sect. 6.5.

Some projects require the use of qualitative methods such as interviews and/or focus groups to evaluate certain aspects of an educational intervention. These methods are discussed in the book chapter on research.

6.4.4   Statistical Considerations

Sample Size and Power Calculations In some instances, the intended learner population could be quite specific and small. For example, one may be interested in examining the efficacy of a virtual reality simulator in improving senior anesthesiology residents' difficult airway management skills. If there are only ten senior residents in the program, the evaluation would only have five trainees in control and intervention groups. It is crucial to conduct a power analysis to ensure that the evaluation has adequate power. G*Power [9] is an open-source software available for both Windows and Mac users that has the ability to calculate power for a wide variety of tests including t-tests, F-tests, and chi-square tests. It can also display the results graphically.

Data Analysis Before any analyses are carried out, there needs to be clarity around how the data is aggregated to test the model being used. This is known as the unit of

Table 6.2 Kirkpatrick four-step framework for aligning outcomes, intervention, and measurement instruments

Kirkpatrick four-step framework	Outcomes	Intervention	Measures
Reaction	Increased awareness and confidence in applying pain management principles to patient care	Lectures on pain management concepts, principles, and techniques	A posttest self-report survey to measure usefulness and learner satisfaction of the training program
Learning	Increased knowledge and skills for effective pain management	Hands-on training workshop program involving standardized patients and simulation-based deliberate practice to improve procedural skills applying pain management techniques	A knowledge test and skill checklist administered before and after the intervention
Behavior	Effectively manage pain	Practice patient care skill on actual patients at the postsurgical unit	An observational checklist to measure learners' pain management skills during actual patient encounters
Results	Patients receive better pain management	Practice patient care skill on actual patients at the postsurgical unit; emphasis will be placed on pain management and use of trained interventions	Patients will be surveyed about their post-surgery pain levels and satisfaction. A historical control will be used as a comparison to examine any improvements in the patient outcomes

analysis and is guided by the research question. For example, in the scenario above looking at anesthesia resident airway management skills, the unit of analysis for improvement could be measured at the level of the individual learner or data might be aggregated as residents in different cohort years or as cohorts in different residency programs.

For questionnaires with Likert-scale items, it is necessary to check normal distribution (i.e., using Shapiro–Wilk test, etc.). However, Likert-scale items are often skewed and rarely normally distributed. These data can be analyzed using nonparametric tests. For example, for a single-group pretest–posttest design, a Wilcoxon signed-rank test, and for a control-group pretest-posttest design, a Mann–Whitney U test can be used to analyze group differences. Typically, such data are also reported as frequencies and percentages and represented in tables or bar charts.

Knowledge tests with multiple-choice questions can often produce numerical data calculated as percent correct for each learner and can be analyzed using parametric tests (t-test or ANOVA, etc.) if assumptions are met. It is often necessary to report item analyses including the difficulty and discrimination indices for a knowledge test using the pretest responses. Item difficulty indicates the percentage of test-takers answering a given item correctly. As a frame of reference, for a true/false item, 80–85%, and for a five-response (a, b, c, d, e) item, 65–70% are an ideal difficulty. Item discrimination indicates how well a test item discriminates between individuals who receive high scores on the overall test versus those who scored low. As for the discrimination indices, typically 0.30 and above (up to 1.00) is good while a value between 0.10 and 0.30 is fair. A zero means no discrimination between high- and low-scoring individuals, and a negative value means that those participants who scored high on the entire test answered this question wrong yet those who scored much lower on the test were more likely to get the correct answer.

6.4.5 *Ethical Considerations*

In evaluation, considerations of ethical issues include but are not limited to the equity of learning opportunity for all students within an educational program when a new curriculum component is offered to a subset of the larger group, offering incentives—gift cards, food, or education credits—in exchange for participation, an evaluator being in an authority role (or perceived to have influence over a participant). These factors and any other issues posing a potential for coercion or undue influence for selection/response can cause bias in the study. A more in-depth discussion of the ethical considerations can be found in this book's chapter on ethics.

6.5 Action/Implementation

At this stage, the outcomes and assessment tools are already aligned, and previously published instruments are gathered for evaluating a given scholarship project. Sometimes, it becomes necessary to construct instruments such as questionnaires, checklists, rubrics, knowledge tests, interview/focus group protocols, and coding schemes. The steps taken to construct an assessment tool (i.e., literature review, Delphi technique, cognitive interviews, pilot tests) should be clearly reported in the methods section of a manuscript. There are some resources that provide clear guidance on how to develop high-quality questionnaires [10]. After instruments are developed, a pilot test may be necessary to:

- Determine the reliability and validity of an instrument,
- Check knowledge test item difficulty and discrimination,
- Gauge whether a questionnaire is clear and concise (cognitive interview),
- Train and calibrate raters.

6.5.1 Considerations for Validity and Reliability

Establishing measurement quality is an important step in building a compelling argument for the merits of a given scholarly project and dissemination. Even when using published instruments, one still needs to examine the measures with the target learner population in the context of a specific project. For example, a measure found to produce reliable and valid results with senior medical students in a rural health care setting may not produce similar results with internal medicine residents at a large academic center.

Reliability: Reliability is the consistency or reproducibility of the scores produced by a given assessment tool. There could be several different ways to examine the reliability of scores depending on the type of measure used and the assessment context.

- *Internal consistency:* Internal consistency may be important for a knowledge test or a questionnaire intended to measure a single construct. This means that responses to each item on the assessment tool have a high correlation with one another. Typically, two types of tests are used to examine this, Cronbach's alpha or Kuder-Richardson 20 (KR-20). For instruments using a binary scale (yes/no or correct/incorrect), these two tests basically produce identical results. However, for Likert scales (as in questionnaires with a 5-point scale from "1 = strongly disagree" to "5 = strongly agree," etc.), Cronbach's alpha is more appropriate. Low internal consistency may indicate that the tool could be measuring more than one construct. If the goal is to combine scores from all the questions of a questionnaire into a composite score (e.g., resident burnout score) to use in evaluation analysis, then a factor analysis may be required to examine the factor structure of the questionnaire. This process could help flag the questions that do not seem to be measuring the same construct as the rest of the tool.
- *Test-retest or reproducibility:* Test-retest reliability examines whether an assessment tool is producing consistent scores across different time points using the same individuals. For example, if responses to the assessment tool by the same individuals change drastically from Monday to Friday of the same week with no intervention in between, then this tool may not be reliable to use for evaluation purposes.
- *Interrater reliability*: When multiple raters use a checklist or a rubric to measure procedural skills or communication skills, it will be critical to examine to what extent scores assigned by different raters on the same individuals/performance are consistent. The use of clear descriptors explaining what performance looks like at each different level included in the checklist/rubric and the use of a calibration process often help increase interrater reliability. Calibration process typically involves all raters independently using a checklist/rubric to score a few representative performances and then together examining and resolving discrepancies in their scores. This process helps raters to consistently apply the assessment tool.

- *Generalizability theory:* In any measurement situation, there may be more than one source of variance that is observed in the scores. Typically, the assumption is that the variation in scores represents the true difference in the learners' levels of knowledge or skills. However, as discussed previously, different raters can score the same individuals differently. Likewise, several other factors (called facets) can contribute to the variance in scores as well. For example, different facets that can cause variance in the scores for a given assessment tool include the items/questions/tasks, the time that the assessment is administered, or any other measurement conditions that are considered. This makes it challenging to use a single score to depict the true skill of a learner; in other words, a single score might not be sufficient to generalize to a learner's overall performance when all other factors are considered. For example, when measuring a resident's communication skills in a simulated environment, the simulation scenario, the clinical team composition, and/or the actual standardized patient can all make a difference in how the trainee performs. Generalizability theory or G-theory is useful in such situations to examine multiple sources of variance and their interactions. Typically, including multiple observations (e.g., simulated scenarios) and using multiple raters increase the chances of the scores depicting the actual skills of the trainees.

Reliability is required for an assessment tool to produce good data for evaluation purposes, but it is insufficient or would not imply validity. For example, a knowledge test on anaphylaxis including several MCQs on the etiology and pathophysiology may produce consistent scores across occasions and target learners but may not effectively measure the actual outcome of interest—to recognize atypical anaphylaxis and identify the correct route and location of administration. Therefore, those who receive high scores on this test may or may not actually perform well in a simulated anaphylactic shock scenario. Validity is required for making valid interpretations based on evaluation results.

Validity: Validity is not an inherent quality of an assessment tool; rather, it has to do with the interpretations and implications derived from the scores it produces [11]. This means that an assessment tool is not valid but the scores it produces can be. For compelling evaluation results, validity evidence should be established for each scholarship project [12]. There are several different sources from which validity evidence can be collected. These are the content, response process, internal structure, correlation to other similar measures, and consequences of scores. It may not be feasible or even needed for each specific assessment tool to have all these sources of evidence presented, but often multiple sources should be considered.

- *Content:* The items in an assessment tool should represent the construct (knowledge, skill, or attitude of interest). If the actual construct is not well understood or described, the measurement will not be accurate. For example, multiple-choice questions included in a knowledge test should represent all of the content in a balanced manner. Similarly, a checklist for evaluating advanced trainees' management of blunt abdominal trauma patients should include all critical actions. A literature review often helps explore the different aspects of the construct. An assessment tool can be drafted based on the literature search. However, other methods such as Delphi technique and/or cognitive task analysis may be needed to finalize the actual content of the assessment tool. A detailed description of the process followed should be provided for content evidence.

- *Delphi technique:* This is an iterative process that can be used for reaching a consensus to finalize an assessment tool based on a panel of experts. In multiple rounds, the experts vote to indicate what is essential to include in the assessment tool. After each round, experts receive a summary of results for inclusion or exclusion and are asked to revote for undetermined elements of the instrument. The process ends once experts reach a consensus or some predefined agreement threshold that all pertinent aspects of the construct are represented in the instrument and irrelevant ones are removed. A fair question would be whether the results would differ if different experts were to be included. Therefore, a rationale should be provided for expert selection decisions.
- *Cognitive task analysis:* For complex tasks, a simple observation may not be sufficient to identify all the critical steps needed for successful task completion. Cognitive task analysis can help reveal the underlying decision-making process that is not accessible to direct observation. This method may be needed to understand how an expert thinks by identifying cognitive activities required for a task. This is critical especially for developing checklists to measure performance on complex medical procedures.

- *Response process*: It is critical for an assessment process to represent the real-life behavior that is expected of learners. For example, a knowledge test may not be the most authentic assessment to measure an internal medicine residents' diagnostic ability, but a chart-stimulated recall (a structured interview exploring problem-solving by reviewing patient charts) may be more appropriate. The closer the response behavior during the assessment to real-life settings, the easier it will be to defend the interpretations and implications of the scores.
- *Internal structure*: As mentioned in the internal consistency, examining the factor structure of an assessment tool is important especially if composite scores are meant to be used for decision-making or analysis.
- *Correlation to other similar measures*: If there are similar instruments measuring the same construct, it may be useful to administer them and provide evidence as to what extent scores based on each instrument correlate with one another. This is especially crucial if a newly developed questionnaire or a knowledge test is being used for evaluation.
- *Consequences of scores*: Ultimately, it is critical for any assessment tool to produce actionable data. Consequence validity evidence refers to how the scores produced by an instrument are used and what positive or negative impact that

would have on the learners. For example, if a knowledge test shows a consistent knowledge gap for a certain topic concept, then more instruction should help address this. Consequences of the scores are the intended use of the results. This type of evidence is the least frequently reported in publications; however, careful consideration should be given to discuss what intended and unintended consequences an assessment tool may have had.

Reflection in action: After the pilot test, assessment tools can be revised further before data collection begins for the evaluation.

6.6 Analysis

Following are some steps for analyzing the data for evaluation
- Examine data quality, missing data, and outliers.
- Determine how to handle missing data (despite the best evaluation design, intentions, and efforts, one will face the challenges of dealing with missing or incomplete data in educational evaluation).
- Develop tables and/or figures for descriptive data (demographics, responses to Likert-scale items).
- Examine assumptions for parametric tests.
- Run statistical tests.

6.7 Conclusion

As a key aspect of a scholarly project, evaluation efforts are interwoven throughout the project from inception to reporting. In this chapter, several relevant concepts, evaluation design considerations, and frameworks have been discussed. These should help provide some guidance for planning and executing a robust evaluation. Reporting the evaluation results is also an important undertaking. It may be a daunting task to digest the evaluation results and reflect back on all evaluation efforts as a whole and synthesize them relative to the rest of the scholarly project. Evaluation is a costly enterprise in terms of required time and resources. Thus, it deserves all the time it takes to write a high-quality evaluation report and reflective discussion. It is possible to feel tired at the end of all evaluation activities, and it could be tempting to write this final section rather hastily. However, for a compelling argument that a given scholarship project makes a meaningful contribution to the field, a comprehensive and concise synthesis and discussion need to tie everything together. How to write for publication as well as how to frame your scholarship project for dissemination are given consideration in detail in the following chapters.

6.8 Questions

Discussion Questions

1. What is the importance of evaluation in a scholarly project?
2. What are some evaluation frameworks that can be used in educational scholarship, and how would they help you with your own educational project?
3. How can evaluation results be used to build a compelling argument for the merits of a given scholarly project, and what are some examples of effective strategies for doing so?
4. What are some emerging trends and innovations in educational evaluation, and how might they impact the future of educational scholarship?

Activities

1. Design an evaluation plan for your educational scholarship project. Include the following:

   (a) An evaluation framework
   (b) Research questions
   (c) Learning outcomes
   (d) Evaluation design
   (e) Measures

References

1. Kuhn TS. The structure of scientific revolutions. 2nd ed. Chicago: The University of Chicago Press; 1970.
2. Krathwohl DR. A revision of Bloom's taxonomy: an overview. Theory Pract. 2002;41(4):212–8.
3. Miller GE. The assessment of clinical skills/competence/performance. Acad Med. 1990;65(9):S63–7.
4. Kirkpatrick DL. The four levels of evaluation: measurement and evaluation. Alexandria: American Society for Training and Development; 2007.
5. Lindeman BM, Lipsett PA. Curriculum development for medical education: a six-step approach. In: Thomas PA, Kern DE, Hughes MT, Chen BY, editors. Curriculum development for medical education: a six-step approach. 3rd ed. Baltimore: Johns Hopkins University Press; 2016. p. 121–67.
6. Varpio L, MacLeod A. Philosophy of science series: harnessing the multidisciplinary edge effect by exploring paradigms, ontologies, epistemologies, axiologies, and methodologies. Acad Med. 2020;95(5):686–9.
7. Anderson LW, Krathwohl DR. A taxonomy for learning, teaching, and assessing: a revision of Bloom's taxonomy of educational objectives. London: Longman; 2001.
8. Thomas PA, Kern DE, Hughes MT, Chen BY, editors. Curriculum development for medical education: a six-step approach. 3rd ed. Baltimore: Johns Hopkins University Press; 2016.
9. Erdfelder E, Faul F, Buchner A. GPOWER: a general power analysis program. Behav Res Methods Instrum Comput. 1996;28:1–11.

10. Artino AR Jr, La Rochelle JS, Dezee KJ, Gehlbach H. Developing questionnaires for educational research: AMEE Guide no. 87. Med Teach. 2014;36(6):463–74.
11. Messick S. Validity of psychological assessment: validation of inferences from persons' responses and performances as scientific inquiry into score meaning. Am Psychol. 1995;50(9):741.
12. Cook DA, Beckman TJ. Current concepts in validity and reliability for psychometric instruments: theory and application. Am J Med. 2006;119(2):e167–6.

Chapter 7
Outcomes of Medical Education Scholarship

Halah Ibrahim and Sawsan Abdel-Razig

7.1 Introduction

The primary goal of medical education is to produce…high-quality health care. […] There has been, however, remarkably little investment into the conceptualization and study of the association between the process of medical education and quality of care [14].

In an educational intervention, variables are used to describe both the intervention that occurs in an educational system and the changes that result from the intervention. The *independent variable* (x) is used to denote what causes the change, and the *dependent variable* (y) is used to denote what is expected to change. Outcomes measure the dependent variable (y), the change that occurs as a result of teaching and learning. Determining outcome variables should be an early step in the design of an educational research project. It requires reflection back on the research question and the theoretical framework. One of the most important foundational principles is to make sure the research question and methods align with the selected outcome measures. The best outcome is the one that best answers the research question. The outcome then informs the methodology. The alignment between these three areas is critical to the successful dissemination of the work (Fig. 7.1).

H. Ibrahim (✉)
Department of Medicine, Khalifa University College of Medicine and Health Sciences, Abu Dhabi, United Arab Emirates
e-mail: halah.ibrahim@ku.ac.ae

S. Abdel-Razig
Department of Medicine, Cleveland Clinic Abu Dhabi, Abu Dhabi, United Arab Emirates
e-mail: razigs@clevelandclinicabudhabi.ae

A. S. Fitzgerald, G. Bosch (eds.), *Education Scholarship in Healthcare*,
https://doi.org/10.1007/978-3-031-38534-6_7

Fig. 7.1 Alignment of research question, methodology, and outcome measure

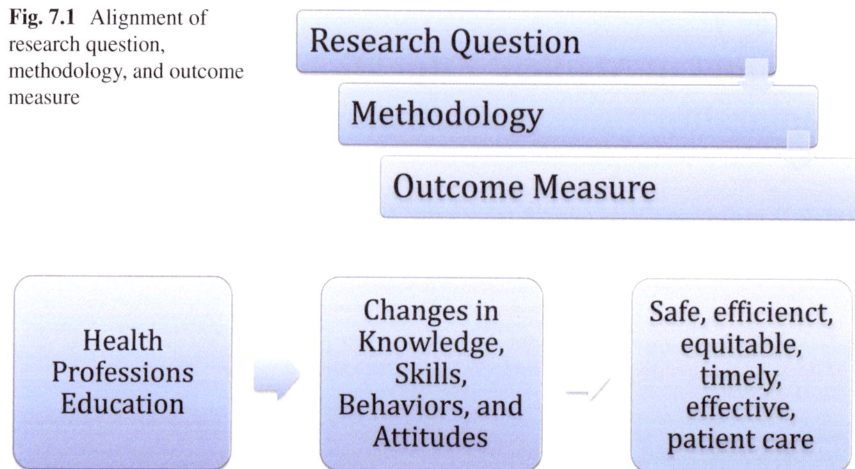

Fig. 7.2 Why outcomes matter in health professions education [14]

7.2 The Benefits of Research Outcomes

We should consider the impact of educational research in the same way that we view the impact of clinical research. As the outcomes of clinical research inform our clinical practice, the outcomes of educational research should inform our educational practice. Well-designed education research can, therefore, provide evidence-based guidance for decision-making in health professions education.

For example, the flipped classroom has been shown to promote higher-order thinking in nursing education [1], and active learning, such as the flipped classroom, has been shown to improve learning and course performance [2]. These findings have prompted many nursing programs to adopt the flipped classroom model (Fig. 7.2).

Outcomes of medical education research address information that is important to the assessment of learners and instructors, and they also provide critical information to the institution and the program. Therefore, the constituents in medical education include the learners, faculty, educational programs, institutions, patients, and the larger society.

7.3 Defining the Unit of Analysis

The study population in medical education usually involves trainees, faculty, health-care workers, and patients. The evaluation outcomes of these study populations can be measured at various levels of aggregation or disaggregation. These levels are sometimes referred to as the unit of analysis [3].

Common units of analysis in medical education research
- Individual—e.g., first-year nursing student
- Institution—e.g., a cohort of pharmacy students at a single institution
- System—e.g., all dialysis patients in a healthcare system
- Geographic—e.g., medical students in the Southeast Region of the United States

It is important to recognize that outcomes at one level might not be generalizable to other levels [4]. For example, educational outcomes in a cohort of nursing students at a single institution might not be generalizable to all nursing students.

7.4   Question—Method—Outcome Alignment

A variable is any entity that can vary by taking on multiple values. Variables are part of research questions. The research question aligns with the problem and purpose and the variable is part of the *Population/Participants (P)*, *Intervention/Independent Variable (I)*, *Comparison (C)*, *and Outcomes (O)* framework we used in this book to write the question.

Once we have identified a research question, we need to decide what research method is most appropriate and then make sure the outcome measures align. First, consider what the outcome (dependent variable) is that you are interested in measuring. Then, consider how it will be operationalized. By operationalize, we mean selecting a metric that represents the outcome of interest.

Example Q1 from Table 7.1: Descriptive Quantitative Research Question—*What is the distribution of scores for internal medicine examinees on the ABIM recertification exam?*

This question is in the format of P—O (Population—Outcomes). There is no intervention, variable, or comparison group.

Method: In this case, the outcome is operationalized by looking at the distribution of test scores as a surrogate for knowledge. An appropriate method would be the statistical analysis of scores. This is an example of learner performance as an outcome. Further research would be needed to assess if there is a relationship between ABIM scores and patient outcomes.

Is there alignment between the Question, Method, and Outcome? Yes, the question asks about examinees taking a recertification examination. The method is a statistical analysis, which is consistent with the question to give the outcome of exam score distributions.

Question: P--O Examinees -- Scores	Method: Quantitative - Statistical Analysis	Outcome: Exam Score Distribution

Table 7.1 Research question frameworks and examples using ABIM/examinees

	Questions	Framework	Generic Template	Example
Example Q1	*Descriptive Quantitative*	P--O	**What is the** outcome **of** participants **on** descriptor?	**What is the** distribution of scores **for** internal medicine examinees **on the** ABIM recertification exam?
	Predictive Quantitative	PI-O	**Does** intervention **affect** outcome **in** population/participant?	**Does** taking a review course **affect** the ABIM exam pass rate **in** recertification examinees?
Example Q2	*Causal Quantitative*	PICO	**Does** intervention **have** outcome **on** population/participant **compared with** comparison group?	**Does** maintenance of certification participation **lead to** higher scores on recertification testing **for** internal medicine examinees **compared to** those who don't participate?
		PICOT	**In** population **does** intervention **compared with** control **cause** outcome **within** timeframe?	**In** internal medicine examinees, **does** a review course **compared with** independent study **affect** the pass rate on the ABIM exam **when** the review course is within 6 months of the exam?
Example Q3	*Qualitative*	PPhTS	**For** participants, **what is** their central Phenomenon, **during** time in space?	**For** ABIM recertification examinees, **what is their** perception of overall burden of testing **during** their most recent test experience in the new home format?

Example Q2 from Table 7.1: Causal Quantitative Research Question—*Does maintenance of certification participation lead to higher scores on recertification testing for internal medicine examinees compared to those who don't participate?*

This question is in the format of PICO (Population—Intervention—Comparison—Outcomes).

Method: This example is similar to the prior example but would require more statistical analysis due to the intervention comparison group.

Is there alignment between the Question, Method, and Outcome? Yes, the question asks about an intervention on a group. The method of quantitative statistical analysis is consistent with the question to give the outcome of comparison.

Question: P-I-C-O Examinees - Intervention - Comparison - Outcome	Method: Quantitaive - Statistical Analysis	Outcome: Comparison - Exam Score Distribution

Example Q3 from Table 7.1: Qualitative Research Question—*For ABIM recertification examinees, what is their perception of overall burden of testing during their most recent test experience in the new home format?*

This question is in the format of PPhTS (Population—Phenomenon—Time—Space).

Method: This type of question is qualitative. The most appropriate methodology should be non-numerical, such as words from interviews, focus groups, or observations.

Is there alignment between the Question, Method, and Outcome? Yes, the outcome in qualitative studies tend to be interpretations, inferences, or themes. In this case, the outcome is perception, namely the perception of burden.

Question: P-Ph-T-S Examinees - Perception - Test Experience - Format	Method: Qualitative - Focus groups	Outcome: Perception of Burden

Let's look at a question not in our table.

Example Q4: Research Question—*Does a faculty development curriculum on feedback lead to improved quality of faculty feedback to trainees?*

First, determine what type of research question. Looking at Table 7.1, we see the question is asking about an intervention (faculty development curriculum on feedback) and an outcome (improved quality of faculty feedback) impacting a population (trainees). The question has the components of Population—Intervention—Outcome, so it appears to be Predictive Quantitative.

Method: There are several methods that could potentially be used to evaluate this study question depending on the outcome of interest. The key to determining what best fits is determining what is meant by improvement. If you are looking at a correlation between attendance in the faculty development curriculum sessions and feedback delivery, the study should be carried out as a relationship study. Perhaps you are interested to see if the faculty who participated in the curriculum had better teaching evaluations than they did in the year prior. That would be a comparison, and the study should be carried out with in with a methodology that compares each faculty member's evaluations before and after the intervention.

Is there alignment between the Question, Method, and Outcome? Yes, the question asks about a faculty development program but has no comparison group. The method is quantitative and gives an outcome that is a correlation regarding improved quality.

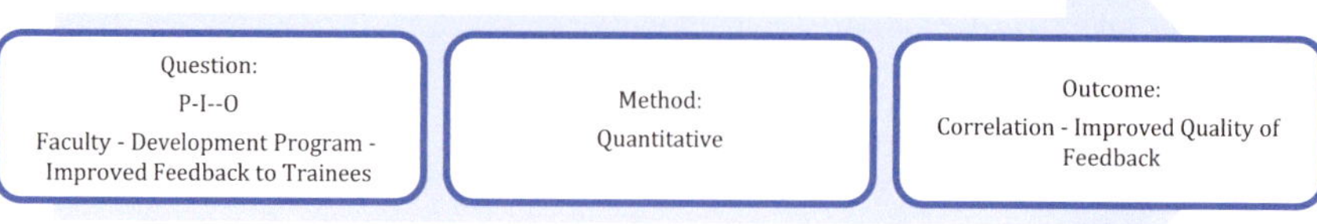

However, it would be a flaw in logic to say that the faculty development program was causal in improving the faculty feedback.

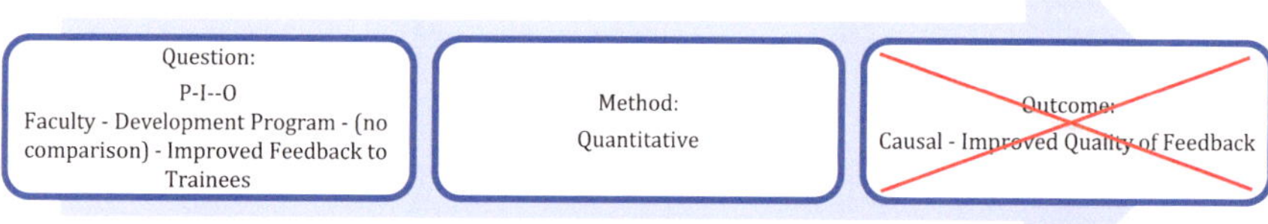

In order to make a statement of outcome causation, the method would need to match the outcome with a more rigorous design that includes a comparison group. One group could be randomized to receive training and one group randomized not to receive training.

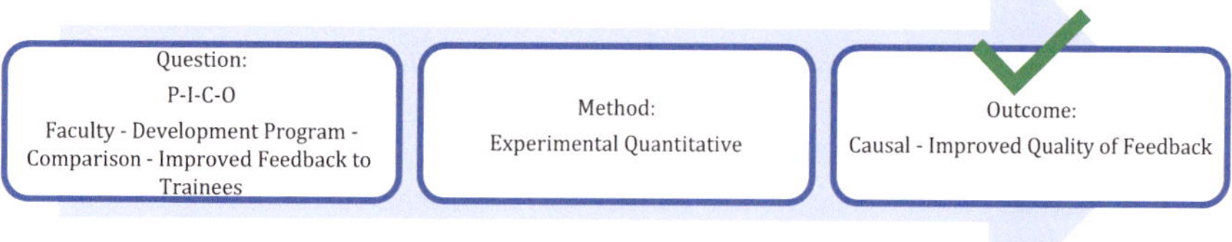

Considerations regarding a research question require thinking about the design of your study and what resources you have. Considerations include the time, manpower, and equipment needed for data collection, analysis, and dissemination of results. Equipment needs might include access to participants, the feasibility of doing a randomized controlled design, computer software for tracking, storing, or analyzing the outcomes measures, and facility workspaces. Additional thoughts on funding sources for these types of additional considerations can be found in this book's Support Chapter.

7.5 Considering Outcomes with Relation to Evaluation Models

With the question-methods-outcomes aligned, the health scholar should consider how evaluation models can help demonstrate the impact of the study results. It is important to choose a model that is congruent with the research question and is logistically feasible to address. Also, when selecting the evaluation design, the researcher should optimize both internal validity and external generalizability of study results. This requires a critical analysis of the study design's strengths and limitations, with special consideration of potential threats to validity, such as biases, measurement, and statistical errors.

Kirkpatrick Training Evaluation Model—The Kirkpatrick Model was designed to objectively measure the effectiveness of training and educational programs [6]. Kirkpatrick's model assesses the effectiveness of educational interventions at four hierarchal levels of program outcomes: (1) learner satisfaction or reaction to the program; (2) learning outcomes attributed to the program (e.g., attitudes changed, knowledge gained, skills improved); (3) changes in learner behavior in the context in which they are being trained (whether the learning transferred into practice in the workplace); and (4) the program's final results (the ultimate impact of training).

Example Q4 (from above): Research Question—*Does a faculty development curriculum on feedback lead to improved quality of faculty feedback to trainees?*

- Kirkpatrick Level 1 (Reaction): Do the participants feel as though they learned effectively from the curriculum?
- Kirkpatrick Level 2 (Learning): Do the participants know how to practice effective feedback delivery?
- Kirkpatrick Level 3 (Behavior): Are the participants using feedback skills in practice?
- Kirkpatrick Level 4 (Results): Has the quality of feedback improved?

Kirkpatrick's model has been criticized for its assumption of causality between the educational program and its outcomes. It also does not take into account the intervening factors that can affect learning, such as learner motivation or the hidden curriculum [7]. However, the model provides a useful taxonomy of outcomes for medical education scholarship (Fig. 7.3).

Miller's Clinical Competency Pyramid—Miller's Pyramid model divides the development of clinical competence into four, hierarchical processes [8]. On the lowest level of the pyramid is knowledge. The next tier represents the application of knowledge. The third level stands for clinical skills competency. Finally, the top level of the pyramid is clinical performance. The lower tiers of the pyramid encompass the cognitive components of competence and can be assessed in the classroom setting; whereas the higher levels assess behavioral components of clinical competence, often assessed in simulated and real-world clinical settings.

Example Q4 (from above): Research Question—*Does a faculty development curriculum on feedback lead to improved quality of faculty feedback to trainees?*

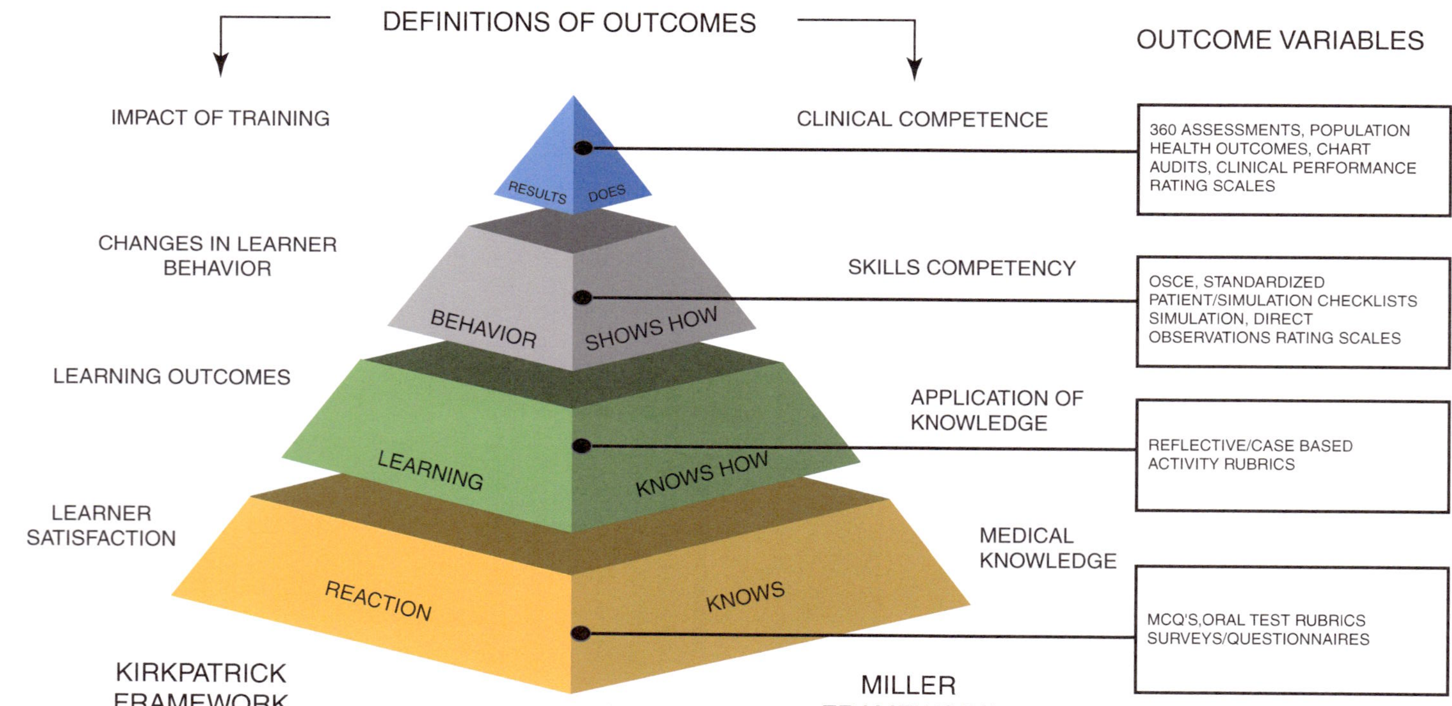

Fig. 7.3 Miller and Kirkpatrick evaluation models and related outcome variables

- Miller's Level 1 (Knows): Does the learner possess an appropriate knowledge base?
- Miller's Level 2 (Knows How): Can the faculty member explain how they will provide feedback?
- Miller's Level 3 (Shows How): Can the faculty member provide feedback effectively when prompted, such as during role-play?
- Miller's Level 4 (Does): How well does the faculty member provide feedback in their daily practice?

Moore's Expanded Learner Outcomes—Moore Jr et al. [9] proposed an expanded model of learning, specifically in response to the concept of continuous learning required in the health professions and a need to integrate assessment, planning, and outcomes. In this framework, Moore combined a continuing medical education (CME) framework with Miller's Pyramid (Fig. 7.4).

Example Q4 (from above): Research Question—*Does a faculty development curriculum on feedback lead to improved quality of faculty feedback to trainees?*

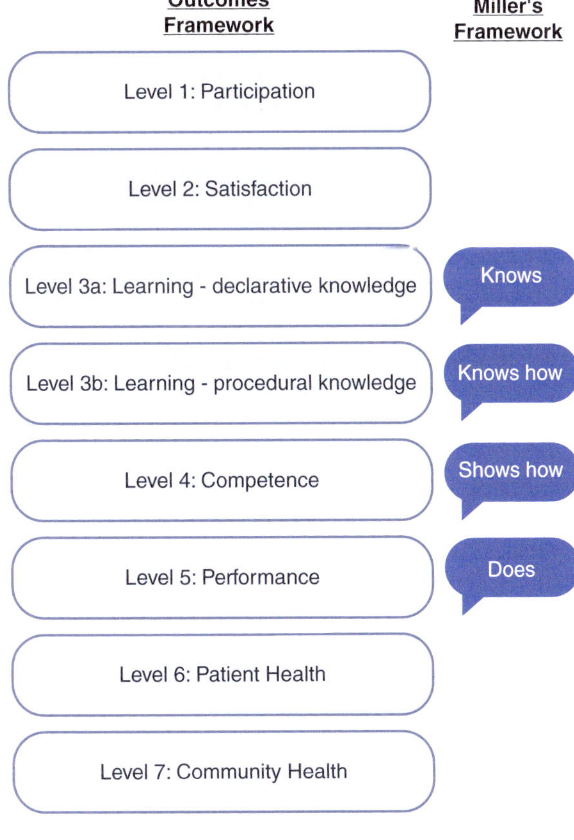

Fig. 7.4 Moore's expanded learner outcomes*

*Moore, Greene, & Gallis, 2009

- Moore's Level 1 Participation: Did the learners attend and actively participate?
- Moore's Level 2 Satisfaction: Did the learners feel actively engaged?
- Moore's Level 3a Learning-declarative knowledge [Knows]: Does the learner possess an appropriate knowledge base?
- Moore's Level 3b Learning-procedural knowledge [Knows How]: Can the faculty member tell you they will provide feedback?
- Moore's Level 4 Competence [Shows How]: Can the faculty member provide feedback effectively when prompted?
- Moore's Level 5 Performance [Does]: How well does the faculty member provide feedback in their daily practice?
- Moore's Level 6 Patient Health: Do trainees perceive feedback training has helped them to improve patient care?
- Moore's Level 7 Community Health: Has feedback culture within the institution improved?

The levels to measure depend on the feasibility of the study and the existing literature. If the literature review reveals published studies that address Kirkpatrick and/or Miller level 1–2, conducting a similar study with the same outcome measures is less likely to be of interest to journal editors. It would then be wise to consider targeting higher level outcomes if those outcomes are a gap in the literature. Alternatively, if you are exploring an entirely new area where even the understanding of learner reaction is novel and would address a gap in the literature, then a robust measure of that level would be potentially interesting to education journals and their readers. Many educational scholarship studies measure multiple different levels, and by measuring at different levels, you get a better idea of the effectiveness of your intervention.

In addition to ensuring that outcome variables are appropriate, address the study question, align with study design and methods, and use a specified evaluation models, a critical consideration in rigorous educational scholarship is the determination of the validity of measurement—that is how accurately a specific outcome variable measures the intended educational construct.

Most educational scholarship involves the use or development of evaluation instruments for the various study participant groups (learners, institutions, or systems). Medical educators recognize the importance of reliable and valid teaching assessments [10]. Yet, consistent validity criteria are not always employed when developing and assessing instruments used in clinical teaching [11]. At each level of outcomes, educational health scholars must consider the validity evidence of the instruments being developed or used to measure the specified outcome.

The five-category validity framework, introduced by Messick, has been widely used in medical education research [12]. In this best practice approach, the five sources of validity evidence include: (1) Content, (2) Response Process, (3) Internal Structure, (4) Relation to Other Variables, and (5) Consequences.

In general, quantitative instruments such as multiple-choice question examinations or surveys are more amenable to rigorous content validity, though they may represent the lowest evaluation paradigm (knows/reaction level), whereas outcomes at the highest level of impact (does/impact of training) may use instruments with considerably lower construct validity evidence (e.g., 360° assessments or chart audits). Figure 7.5 superimposes the current state of validity evidence in health professions education literature across the various levels of outcomes.

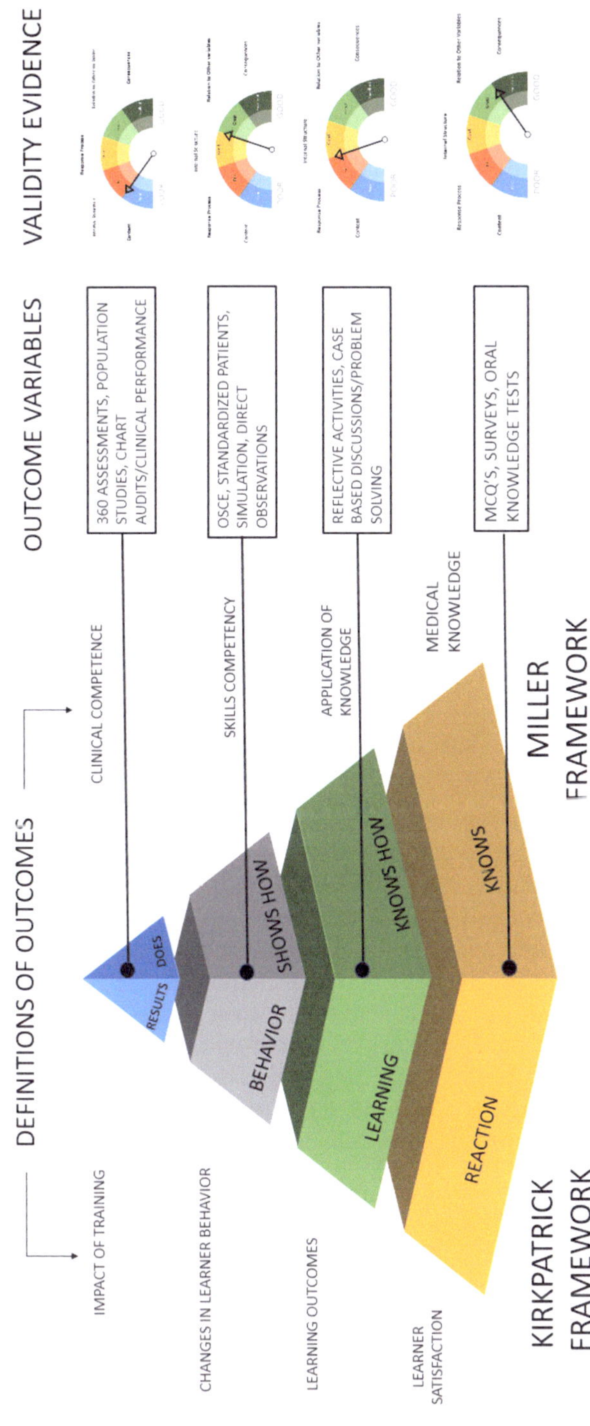

Fig. 7.5 Miller and Kirkpatrick models, outcome variables, and evidence of validity

Table 7.2 Selecting specific outcome measures

Outcome measure	Measure	Miller's level	Kirkpatrick's level
Performance audit	Performance, skill	4	4
Direct observation	Performance, skill	3 or 4	3
Global rating scale[a]	All	3 or 4	3 or 4
Reflective essay	Attitudes	2	2 or 3
Oral examination	Knowledge, attitudes	2 or 3	2 or 3
Written examination	Knowledge	1 or 2	2 (usually)
Survey/questionnaire	Attitudes, perceptions, process	N/A	1
Self-assessment	Attitudes, perceptions	N/A	1

Adapted from Ryan MS, Quigley PD, Lee CC, Chua I, Paul CR, Gigante J, Beck Dallaghan G. Innovation to Dissemination Workshop: Selecting Outcome Measures to Translate Educational Innovations Into Scholarship. *MedEdPORTAL*. 2018;14:10759 [5]
[a]Subject to rater biases and subjectivity

7.6　Selecting Specific Measures

There are many outcome measures available. However, many of them fall into typical categories. Table 7.2 summarizes the major outcome measures in terms of what each measure in the Miller and Kirkpatrick levels.

7.7　Challenges to Patient Outcomes Research

Over the decades, there have been multiple calls in academic journals for examination of the link between health professions education and the quality of patient outcomes [14]. The reasons to be concerned with patient outcomes are strong—they are important components of Glassick's criteria, and they are the ultimate goal of health professions education. Outcomes commonly used in medical education scholarship are often proximal, such as learner knowledge, performance, satisfaction, and attitude, whereas patient-centered outcomes are evaluated infrequently—in only 0.7% of studies according to a review of the literature performed in 2001 and in 2.3% of health professions education studies according to a literature review conducted 18 years later [13]. Despite the potential benefits, research on patient-centered outcomes of medical education requires greater methodological rigor and is fraught with challenges.

Challenges include [14]
- Sample size—the number of participants in a training program is often inadequate to appropriately power the study.
- Lag time—there is often a considerable lag time between an educational intervention and the actual measurement of patient outcomes.
- Limited generalizability—the wide variability among and between medical schools and postgraduate training programs limits generalizability.

- Confounding variables—there are multiple confounding factors that affect any association between education and clinical outcomes.
- Difficulty showing causality—the outsized impact of individual practice and healthcare systems on patients dilute the ability to demonstrate direct causal links between medical education interventions and patient outcomes.
- Experimental designs limitations

  - Most studies employ non-randomized methodologies, including cross-sectional designs or retrospective studies using historical controls.
  - Most studies do not include genuine control groups for which the educational intervention is delayed or withheld.

7.8 Conclusion

Outcomes of educational interventions usually measure changes in attitudes, knowledge, skills or behaviors of a pre-defined learner group. Outcome variables of education scholarship should be derived directly from the research question and the conceptual paradigm of the study. Congruence between study objectives, outcome variables, methodology and the data collection instrument is critical to ensure the scientific rigor of the medical educator's scholarship. Though the ultimate goal of health professions education research is the development and implementation of educational interventions that positively impact patient or population health metrics, relating educational outcomes at that level is complex and fraught with multiple confounding factors. Nonetheless, through methodical consideration of study question, variable determination, study designs, and outcomes measurement, medical education researchers can advance the value and impact of our discipline and ultimately on healthcare (Fig. 7.6).

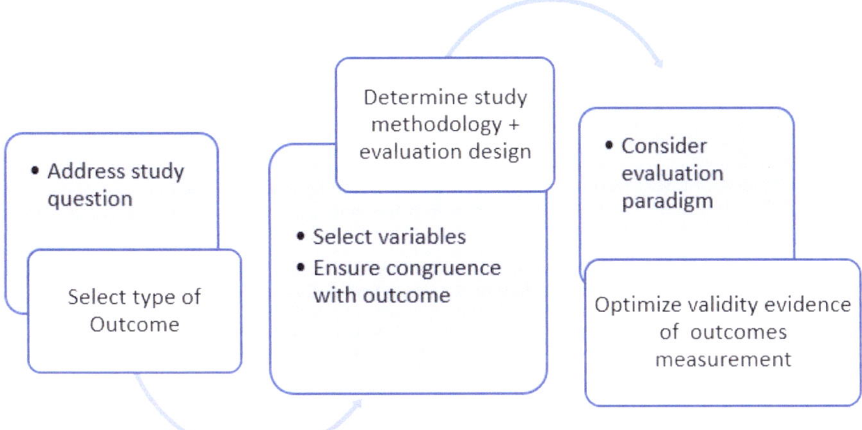

Fig. 7.6 Summary of considerations

7.9 Questions

Activities
1. For your research project, what are the outcomes (dependent variables) that the research question is designed to answer?
2. For each identified variable, what is the unit of analysis that the variable describes?
3. Check the research question, planned methodology, measurement instrument, and outcome measure for your project to ensure that they align.

References

1. Missildine K, Fountain R, Summers L, Gosselin K. Flipping the classroom to improve student performance and satisfaction. J Nurs Educ. 2013;52(10):597–9.
2. Freeman S, Eddy SL, McDonough M, Smith MK, Okoroafor N, Jordt H, Wenderoth MP. Active learning increases student performance in science, engineering, and mathematics. Proc Natl Acad Sci. 2014;111(23):8410–5.
3. Remler DK, Van Ryzin GG. Research methods in practice: strategies for description and causation. Thousand Oaks: Sage Publications; 2021.
4. Prystowsky JB, Bordage G. An outcomes research perspective on medical education: the predominance of trainee assessment and satisfaction. Med Educ. 2001;35(4):331–6.
5. Ryan MS, Quigley PD, Lee CC, Chua I, Paul CR, Gigante J, Beck DG. Innovation to dissemination workshop: selecting outcome measures to translate educational innovations into scholarship. MedEdPORTAL. 2018;14:10759. https://doi.org/10.15766/mep_2374-8265.10759.
6. Kirkpatrick D. Revisiting Kirkpatrick's four-level model. Train Dev. 1996;1:54–9.
7. Holton E. The flawed four-level evaluation model. Hum Res Dev Q. 1996;7:5–21.
8. Miller GE. The assessment of clinical skills/competence/performance. Acad Med. 1990;65:S63–7. https://doi.org/10.1097/00001888-199009000-00045.
9. Moore DE Jr, Green JS, Gallis HA. Achieving desired results and improved outcomes: integrating planning and assessment throughout learning activities. J Contin Educ Heal Prof. 2009;29(1):1–15. https://doi.org/10.1002/chp.20001.
10. Downing SM. Validity on the meaningful interpretation of assessment data. Med Educ. 2003;37:830–7.
11. Beckman TJ, Ghosh AK, Cook DA, Erwin PJ, Mandrekar JN. How reliable are assessments of clinical teaching? A review of the published instruments. J Gen Intern Med. 2004;19:971–7.
12. Messick S. Validity. In: Linn RL, editor. Educational measurement. 3rd ed. Phoenix: Oryx Press; 1993.
13. Emery M, Wolff M, Merritt C, Ellinas H, McHugh D, Zaher M, Gruppen LD. An outcomes research perspective on medical education: has anything changed in the last 18 years? Med Teach. 2022;44(12):1400–7.
14. Chen FM, Bauchner H, Burstin H. A call for outcomes research in medical education. Acad Med. 2004;79(10):955–60. https://doi.org/10.1097/00001888-200410000-00010.

Chapter 8
Ethics and Research

Michael Malinowski and Michael F. Amendola

8.1   Introduction

The environment of educational research and scholarship within most institutions has a level of intensity and scrutiny regarding ethics in scholarly production. Moral issues in educational scholarship are created by the complexity of the roles of researchers as scholars and educators [1]. Often, the conflict for educational scholars is not between right and wrong decisions, but rather right and less right [2]. This is restated as the dilemma of competing demands or, more correctly, competing benefits within education and educational scholarship. As you consider the issues of ethics within educational scholarship, the intent of ethical review is not to prevent educators from deviating off a benevolent path, but instead, the purpose of ethical review is often to provide context, rationale, and peer assessment of the educator's priorities as to which entities, principles, and stakeholder values are being maintained ahead of other priorities. At the center of these activities is ensuring the rights and protections of learners.

The original version of the chapter has been revised. A correction to this chapter can be found at
https://doi.org/10.1007/978-3-031-38534-6_19

M. Malinowski
Division of Vascular Surgery, Medical College of Wisconsin, Milwaukee, WI, USA
e-mail: mmalinowski@mcw.edu

M. F. Amendola (✉)
Division of Vascular Surgery, Virginia Commonwealth University, Richmond, VA, USA

A. S. Fitzgerald, G. Bosch (eds.), *Education Scholarship in Healthcare*,
https://doi.org/10.1007/978-3-031-38534-6_8

8.2 Ethical Constructs

Within educational research, a fundamental requirement is to establish a framework within which to evaluate differing values of stakeholders within the educational relationship. This framework encompasses *teleological*, *external*, and *deontological* constructs.

- *Teleological* view looks directly at the consequences of the action within the educational relationship and the way they provide immediate benefit or harm within the relationship of the educator and learner.
- *External* ethical tradition extends the scope of review beyond the immediate consequences of an action to include potential consequences that are external, far-reaching, and delayed in nature.
- Deontological perspective only judges the act as moral/ethical or immoral/unethical; resultant consequences are immaterial to the ethical nature of the act itself. If poor outcomes result from an ethical act, that outcome is tolerated as a rational result of an ethical action.

The deontological perspective can be extrapolated with Kantian overtones such that all individuals are autonomous. Therefore, individuals can never be treated as a "means to an end" since individuals must always be referred to as their own end [1].

Depending on the ethical tradition being considered, each theory can independently be correct within a comparative framework to the other traditional perspectives because the prioritization of values and the scope of review are different. Likewise, two different traditions can simultaneously determine a single action ethical in one tradition and unethical in another since the foci are dissimilar. Progressing from this understanding that the matrix of ethical considerations and traditions can have similar or adversarial review based on similar conditions within the same scenario, the goal is then to define mechanisms for how to evaluate competing values and stakeholders within educational scholarship.

The philosophical definitions of autonomy, beneficence, non-maleficence, veracity, fidelity, and justice as summarized in the Belmont Report emerged to the forefront of dealing with these complex reviews to ensure a commonality for maintaining valued principles with educational relationships [3]. These conversations are no different from our thoughts within the ethical tradition frameworks. Preservation of individual autonomy within the teaching relationship remains critical to effective adult learning models.

Both beneficence and non-maleficence ensure that the educational event remains a positive and constructive process within the learner's educational career. Fidelity reiterates that all entities are true to intent and adhere to the established "rules" of interaction. Justice is the overall cohesive mechanism dating back to the traditions of Plato, Aquinas, and Mill. For Plato, justice is a virtue that offers rational order [4]. For Aquinas, it is a rational means between opposite sorts of injustices with reciprocal transactions [5]. Mill suggested that justice is a collective name for a plethora of social utilities that protect human liberties [6]. Ultimately, however, the concept of justice is to stabilize entities within society and protect human liberties within the moving parts of social interactions.

8.3 Conflicts of Interest and Power Relationships

For all health scholars, protecting stakeholder ideals and values within appropriate ethical constructs and observation of the need for autonomy and justice are vital. And maintaining the fundamental nature of the teaching relationship within educational scholarship is equally critical. The fidelity and strength of these relationships within educational scenarios are key to appropriate content transmission. Expert educators use trust and adapt to the views, abilities, values, and expectations of their learners to maximize the constructive impact of adult learning. This fiduciary learning relationship occurs explicitly when defining their scope of teaching practice as well as when espousing the ideals, practices, and approaches for the endeavors that support adult learning.

8.3.1 Is Education a Protected Rights Profession?

A consideration of the educational relationship is whether communication in the teaching realm is considered privileged or public property. Should educators be considered to have protections similar to other professions such as medicine, law, and clergy?

In medicine, a patient's personal information is considered private, and private information is protected to prevent discrimination. If a patient's information was not protected in this manner, a patient might not feel secure in the medical system and might not trust their treating healthcare team to maintain confidentiality. If a patient cannot speak candidly and honestly, substandard treatment can result. Similarly, attorney-client privilege ensures that attorneys can provide appropriate legal advice with a full understanding of their client's situation while ensuring a safe environment for clients. Therefore, a privileged communications claim appears reliant on both the type of information and the purpose of the relationship. Most educators agree that teaching does not remain within the realm of a protected rights profession to the same degree as medicine, law, and clergy.

8.3.2 Is Educational Scholarship Intellectual Property (IP)?

An emerging and defining consideration is whether the fruits of academic labor qualify as intellectual property. If so, this would entitle both educators and learners to certain defined rights and responsibilities regarding the creation, review, dissemination, and use of material. Yet, the primary goal of educational scholarship is usually not to produce intellectual property to generate revenue in engineering, manufacturing, computer science, biomedicine, and the pharma industry. Instead, it has historically kept separated from commercialization to avoid conflicts of interest [7].

The primary goal of educational activities is content transmission within the three domains of knowledge and learning—cognitive, affective, and psychomotor. When we speak of intellectual property (IP), we encompass the full range of the creative output of the human mind. A subset of that output is the scholarship that is disseminated from teaching. The dissemination is generally covered and protected in a subset of IP known as copyright.

8.3.3 Learner Privacy Concerns

Previously, we considered the importance of creating a safe atmosphere for patients to share their history with their healthcare team and for clients to share their legal situation with the legal team. The learning environment is another setting where safety has been shown to be a factor. Many institutions consider the learner population to be "vulnerable," although this is not a universal designation.

Privacy and vulnerability have implications that relate to informed implicit and explicit consent. An educator seeking consent from a learner is inherently in an imbalanced power dynamic with the learner, particularly if the educator is the person who ultimately grades the learner. In analyzing data and when information is disseminated, unless measures are taken, information that was shared as part of the educational process and not meant to be public can find itself revealed to others.

Mitigation strategies to maintain a healthy educator relationship start with anonymizing data. Deidentification within scholarship projects holds two main strengths, to prevent bias within the research analysis and/or bias towards the learner. An educator's separation of power is paramount to allow learner grading and research involvement without any suggestion of impropriety. Even the perception of a link between research involvement and a learner's grade can affect the learner–educator relationship. Therefore, mitigation at every step is imperative. An educator assuming separate roles as either educator or principal investigator can often be critical to prevent this perception as well. Because of these multiple inferred conflicts of interest, oversight of educators within these scholarship roles has increased.

Institutional review boards (IRBs) have moved into this domain on behalf of learners, educators, and institutional reassurance. Although the traditional role of an IRB was to assure government-funded human and animal research adhered to strict ethical codes of conduct [8], IRB review can offer an opportunity for educators to have a peer review process of ethical standards and institutional culture but is not a guarantee or certificate of ethical standards. A confounder might occur when an IRB allows a researcher to proceed under an "exempt" status either due to a minimal harm model or "conducted in established or commonly accepted educational settings, involving normal educational practices," especially when focused on the "effectiveness of or the comparison among institutional techniques, curricula, or classroom management methods" [9]. IRB review does not protect an educational scholarship project from affecting poorer educational outcomes since its primary role is protection from harm in federally funded studies, and an IRB certainly may not be the best entity to determine educational rigor and product.

8.4 Informed Learners

Educators want to be able to teach learners and also conduct an educational scholarship project. Informed consent is critical so educators and learners alike have reassurance about the terms of the relationship. Historically, consent was often implicit—yet, not required and implicit are clearly not the same supposition. Although explicit consent can remind all parties that consent is being obtained, implicit consent does not mean that consent was not. Is implicit consent to an educational scholarship project an inherent agreement between learners and educators if all other tenets are maintained such as maintaining the quality of current education and learner outcomes? If implicit consent is appropriate, then perhaps one of the largest determinants of the implication of that consent is the institutional culture of the creation and maintenance of educational scholarship at that institution.

Explicit consent assumes that a clear response from the learner is required to confirm participation and allows learners to remove themselves from participation. This ability to opt out is different from the default status conferred with implicit consent since learners may not be aware that they have the ability or mechanism to remove themselves from participation in educational scholarship short of removing themselves from the educational activity and relationship itself. Explicit consent, therefore, allows for better informed consent and the option to continue in the educational opportunity without participation in the project.

8.5 Case Examples

Ethics and ethical approaches are best defined and debated in the midst of case studies and examples.

8.5.1 Case Study 1

A general surgeon, Dr. S, has developed a suture-tying curriculum as part of a larger residency training program. This novel teaching instruction not only is valuable to the institution but can also fill a gap in the surgical education literature. Dr. S is interested in disseminating the teaching technique in the simulation and surgical educational literature. To gather evidence supporting the curriculum and its outcomes, Dr. S wants to use a published assessment tool of manual dexterity for surgeons to assess videos of learners tying knots before and after an educational program. To implement the scholarship project, Dr. S submits for expedited IRB approval. The university-based IRB denies approval of the study due to the following concerns: (1) identification of learners based on their skin color, (2) possible inadvertent voice recognition of learners during video recording, and (3) concern that the learners will receive biased ratings when they rotate officially with Dr. S's division for their surgery rotation.

Consider the following questions regarding this case
- What is the role of the IRB in protecting the learner as it pertains to their identity exposure during the video recording?
- Does the IRB's role include influencing the curriculum for these learners?
- Are trainees considered vulnerable populations?
- How do you think Dr. S should proceed in addressing the concerns of the IRB?

The ideal function of the IRB is to oversee and adjudicate potential conflicts and issues that arise from research. In the setting of a research project that will be a distributed finding from the program and potentially published, the IRB has the authority to protect the identity of subjects enrolled in the research study—even if the protection impacts the education of the population being protected.

An IRB's charter commonly does not function for the approval of an educational program as it resides in a larger institutional based curriculum. In this case it is part of a graduate medical educational (GME) training program. Other institutional groups—for example a curriculum community and graduate medical educational advisory group—decide if such a curriculum is reasonable and/or valid within a larger educational effort, e.g., the training of general surgery residents in a healthcare system.

The role for protection of this population resides with these governing bodies as it pertains to educational programs. However, some institutions will designate the learners within their institution to be categorized as vulnerable for purposes of the institutional IRB.

A pathway forward for additional protection of these learners would be to resubmit the project for review with additional protection for the learners. In this case, the learners could wear surgical gloves and a gown to obscure skin color during the film and ensure that the framing does not show the neck/face; the video could be recorded without sound or with the learner's voices altered. To prevent grading bias, learners who participate in the study could be assigned to other attendings or monitoring could be performed of Dr. S's grading to ensure that no bias is evident.

8.5.2 Case Study 2

A pharmacist educator, Dr. P, has several years of experience in teaching and emphasizing to pharmacy students the need for obtaining an adequate medical history for medicine reconciliation as part of patient examinations. Educational materials were developed over several years based on Dr. P's daily clinical practice. As part of this effort, a fellow academic pharmacist encourages Dr. P to develop and implement a 50-question survey to learners regarding their opinions about the program and their impressions of the educational value of the program. Consider the following questions regarding this case:

- Is there a role for seeking approval from an oversight board regarding learners completing the survey?
- What aspect of the survey could be considered intrusive into the learner's educational environment?
- Could survey participation be considered coercive for learners who are rotating with Dr. P?
- Are curriculum process improvement and program evaluation for scholarship the same if they use the same survey?

Whether approval is needed to have students fill out a survey giving their impression of the educational value of Dr. P's teaching depends on the intended use of the information that is gained from the survey. If Dr. P intends to use the information formatively for curriculum improvement, then seeking institutional review board (IRB) approval of the survey is not needed. However, if Dr. P has the intention to publish the results of the survey at any time in the future, then it is prudent to seek IRB approval before implementing the survey.

One way to approach the implementation of a new intervention is to consider the benefits and risk/harms impacting a learner. At first glance, a survey might appear harmless, but a 50-question survey imposes a burden of time and energy. Since the intent of the survey is feedback to Dr. P regarding the value of the curriculum, the learner appears to derive no benefit. Dr. P might want to consider streamlining the survey to just a few key questions to lessen the burden for learners.

Dr. P is in a more senior position relative to the learners, and therefore there is an imbalance of power in the relationship. The learners may be experiencing pressure—even if unintentional—to complete the survey to please their instructor. The power dynamic can be offset partially by anonymizing the survey. Making participation voluntary can help prevent the appearance of or actual connection to learners' grades.

Even if they use the same survey, curriculum process improvement and program evaluation for scholarship are different. If a survey is intended for internal use only in order to help make improvements to a course, it is governed by different rules than the same survey that is gathering information for use in a later publication.

8.5.3   Case Study 3

Dr. ID is an academic pediatric infectious disease doctor who is tasked with training preclinical medical students in an elective course on population medicine. Dr. ID has an upcoming academic promotion board for possible promotion from assistant professor to associate professor, and a key metric in the promotion scoring is in the enrollment in the medical school elective courses. Dr. ID approaches students being taught in the core medical school curriculum and offers extra credit to those who sign up for the population medicine elective course. Dr. ID also advertises the elective course and its merits to current students during office hours and as part of lectures. Consider the following questions regarding this case:

- What values are misaligned in this case?
- Is it okay for Dr. ID to advertise the elective course during the core curriculum?
- Can Dr. ID's section chief help?
- Do you think metrics like increased enrollment are reasonable to measure academic productivity and justification for promotion?

Pressure from the promotion process is causing Dr. ID to value enrollment numbers over the fair grading of students. Pressure for grades is enticing students to choose electives for extra credit rather than based on their interests. Desire for a quantifiable metric for promotion is causing the promotions committee to choose enrollment as a proxy for quality of teaching though it might not be correlated.

Dr. ID should check to see if there are any guidelines already established at the institution by the governing curriculum committee. Advertising during the core curriculum should follow institutional policy and should be without the perception of quid pro quo such as extra credit to students who enroll.

In the near term, if Dr. ID's section chief agrees with advertisement of the elective course, the section chief as well as others in the section could advertise the elective course to help boost enrollment before the upcoming promotion board. As a longer term fix, the section chief could help lobby for a different promotion metric, one that does not use enrollment as a proxy for value.

In this case, Dr. ID is being judged by a metric which in its basis is not the full assessment of academic productivity/scholarship. A better measure for the institution would be a learner-based evaluation of the program to assess the goals, objectives, and effectiveness of the instructor in conveying the essential components of the curriculum to the learner.

8.6   Conclusion

The environment of educational research and scholarship within most institutions of higher learning in the current era is marked by an increased level of intensity and scrutiny regarding ethical demands on faculty, learners, and scholarly production.

Philosophical definitions of autonomy, beneficence, non-maleficence, fidelity, and justice emerge to the forefront of dealing with these complex reviews to ensure that we are maintaining valued principles with the educational relationship.

Informed consent whether by explicit or implicit means is critical so that educators and learners have reassurance about the terms of their trusted relationship. For all health scholars, protecting the ideals and values of stakeholders within appropriate ethical constructs with observation of the needs of autonomy and justice is vital to protect the institutions of education and education scholarship.

8.7 Questions

Activities

1. Considering the readings, identify (1) benefits and (2) potential risks to participants in your own study/project.

    (a) As you consider risks, remember to include burdens imposed by participation in your project such as burden, cognitive load, and opportunity cost of participation.
    (b) Are there ways to further improve the benefits and minimize risks to your project participants?

References

1. Healey RL, Bass T, Caulfield J, Hoffman A, McGinn MK, Miller-Young J, Haigh M. Being ethically minded: practicing the scholarship of teaching and learning in an ethical manner. Teach Learn Inquiry. 2013;1(2):23–33.
2. Badaracco JL Jr. The discipline of building character. Harv Bus Rev. 1998;76(2):114–24.
3. U.S. Department of Health and Human Service, Office for Human Research Protections. The Belmont report. 2016. https://www.hhs.gov/ohrp/regulations-and-policy/belmont-report/index.html.
4. Cooper JM. Plato: complete works. Indianapolis: Hackett; 1997.
5. Regan RJ, Baumgarth WP, Aquinas T, editors. On law, mortality, and politics. Indianapolis: Hackett; 1998.
6. Warnock M, Mill JS, editors. Utilitarianism and other writings. Cleveland: World Publishing Company; 1962.
7. Boyle J, Jenkins J. Intellectual property: law and the information society: case and materials. 5th ed. Durham: Center for Study of the Public Domain; 2021.
8. Code of Federal Regulations, ECFR. 2021. Title 21, chapter 1, subchapter A, Part 56.101.
9. Anderson P. Ethics, institutional review boards and the involvement of human participants in composition research. In: Mortensen P, Kirsch GE, editors. Ethics and representation in qualitative studies of literacy. Urbana: National Council Teachers of English; 1996.

Part IV
Sharing Your Work

Chapter 9
Dissemination

Sean Tackett and David E. Kern

9.1 Introduction

Dissemination is derived from Latin origin with the prefix *dis*-meaning dispersal in all directions and -*sem*- meaning seed [1]. In scholarship, we intend to disseminate facts, ideas, or methods that take root and go on to bear fruit, yielding seeds that might be further disseminated. As you read earlier in the book, dissemination is what turns a scholarly activity into an act of scholarship. Dissemination implies inviting peers to review, incorporating critique, building consensus, and making the improved product available to other scholars and the public to build on further.

9.2 The Benefits of Dissemination

While there can be immediate benefits to dissemination, the power of dissemination occurs over a long timeframe. The ability to record and share knowledge across generations has been an important factor in the evolution of humankind. Technologies that facilitate knowledge sharing (e.g., alphabets and writing, printing press, internet, and mobile devices) have dramatically accelerated innovations that have improved the quality of people's lives. Contributing to the tradition of scholarship by participating in dissemination means that you could be benefitting others for many years to come.

S. Tackett (✉) · D. E. Kern
Johns Hopkins University School of Medicine, Baltimore, MD, USA
e-mail: Stacket1@jhmi.edu; Dkern1@jhmi.edu

© The Author(s), under exclusive license to Springer Nature Switzerland AG 2023

A. S. Fitzgerald, G. Bosch (eds.), *Education Scholarship in Healthcare*, https://doi.org/10.1007/978-3-031-38534-6_9

Besides achieving the long-term goals at the heart of scholarly endeavors, when you disseminate effectively, you can increase your own standing in your field or discipline. When more people know about the work you have done, your credibility and reputation can be enhanced. Colleagues as well as members of the public might be more likely to listen to what you have to say, use the information or resources you provide, share additional feedback that enhances your work, agree to collaborate, or find ways to support you with financial or material resources. It makes sense that academic institutions, which seek to increase their influence over change, commonly have promotion criteria intended to measure your reputation as a scholar.

Dissemination is hard work, so it is important to identify early on what motivates you personally. Dissemination offers an opportunity to draw attention to the problems or interests that made you pursue scholarship in the first place. Taking a moment to remind yourself of the difference you are trying to make by engaging in educational scholarship is a good way to ensure that you achieve what you want when you consider the multitude of dissemination options available to you.

9.3   What to Disseminate?

Scholarship can take a variety of shapes and sizes that blur the lines between traditional concepts of research and education. If you are focusing on research, what you disseminate might be new facts or evidence, or a new theory or framework that was generated during the research process. In this case, you have likely anticipated the scholarly product when formulating your research question.

If you are focusing on program or curriculum development, the program itself— or parts of it—might be what you want to disseminate. If your focus is scholarly teaching, you might disseminate rigorously developed, educational materials.

Ways to think about what to disseminate have been described for health scholars based on Boyer's four forms of scholarship [2, 3]. Examples of publishable products resulting from scholarly work in education have also been described according to Kern's six-step approach for curriculum development in medical education [4] (see Table 9.1).

Table 9.1 illustrates some ways that curriculum development can lead to scholarship. The needs assessments conducted as part of steps 1 and 2 offer opportunities for empiric data collection, e.g., surveys that characterize a health care problem or those given to learners who will participate in the curriculum, or formal literature reviews that synthesize what is known about a given topic. In step 3, goals, objectives, or expected outcomes can be systematically developed through methodologies that build consensus among experts in the field (e.g., through a Delphi process [5]) or key stakeholders for an educational program. Original educational content or innovative educational methods developed for step 4 can be disseminated as reusable learning objects, which are digital curricular units that can be accessed and used across contexts [6]. How a curriculum is implemented (step 5), such as its piloting, how it was adapted to suit a local context, or how barriers were overcome,

Table 9.1 Scholarly products that could be disseminated at different steps of curriculum development

Step in curriculum development	Boyer's forms of scholarship that align most closely with curriculum development step	Examples of educational scholarship
Step 1: Problem identification and general needs assessment	Discovery, integration	Surveys, literature reviews
Step 2: Targeted needs assessment	Discovery, integration	Surveys, interviews, focus groups, literature reviews
Step 3: Goals and objectives	Integration	Standard setting, consensus development (e.g., Delphi method)
Step 4: Educational strategies	Application, teaching	Novel instructional methods, reusable learning objects
Step 5: Implementation	Application, teaching	Case reports on pilots and adaptations
Step 6: Evaluation and feedback	Discovery	Surveys, interviews, focus groups, measurement/scale development
Complete curriculum	Application, teaching	Online curricula, published curriculum manuscripts, curricular repositories (e.g., MedEdPORTAL, MERLOT II)

can provide the basis of a scholarly case report. The measurement instruments developed or data collected during assessment and evaluation in step 6 can often be reported in educational scholarship. Finally, a complete curriculum can be disseminated as a work of scholarship. This can be done online [7], such as in Massive Open Online Courses (MOOCs) or self-paced asynchronous modules, or through online repositories for curricular materials, such as the Association of American Medical Colleges' MedEdPORTAL [8] or the Multimedia Educational Resources for Learning and Online Teaching (MERLOT II) repository [9].

9.4 Where to Disseminate?

There are countless channels and formats for dissemination, and each will have its respective advantages and disadvantages. You should choose what is right for you according to your own goals and the audience that you are trying to reach. For example, those early in an academic career may focus on dissemination channels that are likely to be valued by their institutions or professional organizations, such as peer-reviewed conference submissions or publications. This may enhance their academic reputation and be necessary for career advancement according to promotions criteria. If someone has established academic credibility or is not driven by academic promotion, they might be more interested in less traditional channels and focus on developing online resources, engaging in social media, or using popular mass media outlets. Importantly, dissemination channels and formats are not mutually exclusive, and there can be synergies between them. For example, scholars commonly use their social media presence to amplify work that may be originally published in traditional academic venues. Uploading your work to pre-print archives, such as EdArXiv or bioRxiv, can make the work available to a broad audience and be linked to the publication that has completed the peer-review process.

9.5 Dissemination in Traditional Venues

Detailed advice for common and traditional venues for dissemination is given in upcoming chapters in this book that discuss abstract submissions, poster presentations, and writing peer-reviewed manuscripts. In all of these cases, it is important to be aware of the requirements and conventions of the respective venues. For example, each conference is likely to have its own requirements for abstract submissions that specify formatting and limits on word count. All journals have instructions for authors' sections that detail article format options and other reporting requirements. While not yet required by most journals, it often helps to adhere to reporting guidelines that relate to a specific study design. A useful resource is the Enhancing the Quality of Transparency of health research (EQUATOR) network, which maintains a repository of reporting guidelines [10]. Journals are also bringing greater transparency into the research process. This frequently involves disclosures for all authors and increasingly sharing of specific data collection instruments and deidentified datasets. Some journals are publishing advice for authors [11, 12], descriptions of their peer-review process including competitiveness [13], and reasons for rejection [14]. Finally, it may be useful to consider how an abstract or article publication is indexed by databases, such as Medline, and whether open-access publication is an option, because these factors can impact how easily others can find and access your work.

Textbooks are another traditional venue for dissemination. Textbooks may be more valuable than ever as the sheer quantity of scholarship is becoming overwhelming. Textbooks can curate and integrate a body of content that exceeds the word limit of peer-reviewed manuscripts. Textbooks also give more control to authors to customize a publication of their content and needs. While self-publishing a textbook is becoming more feasible, that process still benefits from working with a professional editor and someone who is familiar with requirements for formatting and publishing books in print or online. Most often, scholars will work with an experienced textbook publisher. This process begins with an author, editor, or team of editors agreeing to terms with a publisher. Then, authors and editors are responsible for generating the content for the book. Editors generally need to identify additional scholars to author specific book chapters. Publishers provide professional formatting of the book and offer the book for sale to individuals and institutional libraries. Sometimes, but not always, royalties from book sales are given to those who contributed to content development. The peer-review process of textbooks is primarily accomplished through the editorial process, although book reviews are sometimes published in academic journals or by academic book review services. Books and their chapters are sometimes indexed in search engines and can generate a citation count.

Mass media outlets such as print journalism or television networks have also been used by scholars to disseminate their work. While engagement is less common for health education scholars, these venues should be considered because they can reach large audiences of experts and nonexperts. You can increase your engagement by connecting with your institution's media specialists and consider preparing a press release. You might also consider proposing an article, short essay, or opinion piece for a newspaper or magazine that draws attention to an issue that matters to you. As we mention below, when disseminating to a broad public audience, it can be important to ensure that you are clearly seeking to discuss the issue at hand rather than seeking to attract publicity for yourself.

9.6   Dissemination in Less Traditional Venues

While Boyer's and Glassick's seminal works remain relevant to scholarship today, they were published before Web 2.0 (which includes wikis and blogs), before mass uptake of social media, and before mobile devices offered information anytime, anywhere. These technologies have revolutionized how we share information of all kinds. They offer opportunities to disseminate the highest quality of information to massive audiences. At the same time, they challenge what it means to have one's work "peer-reviewed" in a manner that meets professional standards.

For example, Wikipedia is one of the most widely used sources for health information in the world and has standards for acceptable contributions. Its articles also undergo quality assurance by designated editors [15]. Yet, Wikipedia has been criticized as a primary source of information [16], and making a scholarly contribution to Wikipedia would likely be given lower status among academic promotions committees than scholarly work disseminated in less read, but more rigorously vetted publications, such as most peer-reviewed journals.

Participating in the creation of reusable learning objects, e.g., instructional videos, or the development of complete online curricula, e.g., in the form of Massive Open Online Courses (MOOCs), can influence large audiences worldwide, but mechanisms of peer review and adjudication are not well established [17, 18].

Scholars can reach many thousands of individuals with reliable content on X (formerly Twitter) or other popular social media platforms. Increasing the quantity of high-quality information on these platforms can serve as a counterweight to the mis- and disinformation spread by others. Scholars themselves can perceive benefits when using social media platforms, such as exposure to new information and learning and formation of new professional connections [19]. What qualifies as scholarship in social media remains contested, although some have proposed guidelines that align with Glassick's criteria [20]. There are also proposed best practices for scholars using social media platforms [19]. Importantly, maintaining your professionalism on social media is a common challenge and requires that all contributions are thoughtful, accurate, and appropriately critical and considerate.

If you intend to develop an original digital resource, such as a podcast (e.g., the popular Key Literature in Medical Education (KeyLIME) Podcast [21]) or a dedicated website (e.g., Must Reads in Medical Education site [22]), you can likewise reach and grow a diverse audience. However, consider that production of these resources will require technical capabilities, and it might take time for a large audience to become aware of the resource.

Preprint archives have been growing in relevance and popularity as the capacity to store information online has increased, and the production of scholarship has accelerated. These archives allow scholars to upload final drafts of manuscripts as they are being submitted to refereed journals and undergoing traditional peer review. They can also store a link to the article once it is published in a journal. Uploaded documents undergo a basic screening for offensive content and plagiarism, and then are publicly available with a corresponding digital object identifier (DOI). Preprints can attract a broader audience than typically encountered by journals and may diversify who is exposed to the content and can give constructive criticism. Published articles that were preceded by a preprint can be cited more often than published articles that did not have a preprint uploaded to an archive [23]. Some view no significant downside to uploading manuscripts to preprint archives [24]. Disadvantages could include that not all journals may be supportive of manuscripts appearing in a preprint archive while undergoing peer review. Moreover, the reliability of the information in preprints may be viewed with skepticism by some researchers [25], and there is an opportunity cost to taking the time to upload manuscripts to preprint archives.

9.7 Dissemination Through Multiple Venues

As Table 9.2 illustrates, there is no single best pathway for dissemination. Each has its respective advantages and disadvantages. Fortunately, you do not need to limit yourself to a single option, and multiple options can complement one another. For example, poster and oral abstract presentations are commonly predecessors for peer-reviewed manuscripts. You could record a teaching activity and disseminate the recording online and on social media. You can use X (formerly Twitter) or other social media to amplify preprints or scholarship published in other venues. Listservs housed by professional organizations or dedicated to health education (e.g., DR-ED listserv for medical education [26]) can be a place to share a variety of scholarly activities with an interested audience and reach those who do not regularly use social media. Because it takes time to establish one's credibility and accrue an audience

Table 9.2 Examples of common channels and formats of dissemination

	Effort in preparation	Competition	Audience size	Audience interaction	Shelf life
Presentations (e.g., institutional or conferences)	+	+	+	+++	+
Workshops	++	+	+	+++	+
Preprints	+++	+	++	++	++
Journal manuscripts	+++	++	++	+	+++
Textbooks	+++	+	++	+	++
Website, wikis, or blogs[a]	+ to +++	+	++	+	++
Social media	+	++	++	++	+
Popular or mass media	+	+++	+++	+	+

[a]Websites, wikis, or blogs can vary considerably in effort required based on the level of customization

(e.g., visitors to a website or followers on social media), engaging in a variety of venues early will allow the best chance for them to complement each other over time.

Finally, as you are considering what venues are most appropriate for your work and your own aspirations, be mindful of the difference between seeking to draw attention to an important issue or problem that motivated your work and promoting yourself or your accomplishments. Most in the scholarly community would acknowledge that passively waiting for others to find one's work amid the vast amount of scholarship (and information in general) competing for attention could limit the work's impact. Most would also support finding ways to enhance the dissemination of scholarly work to reach more people who could use it. However, many scholars also remain sensitive to, and skeptical of, self-promotion, which can signal self-interested motivations and compromise trust. If you are considering broadcasting your work through channels that have large audiences, such as social media, be mindful of how you might be perceived. If in doubt, see if someone can review what you plan to share before you do so broadly.

9.8 Dissemination Resources

Dissemination itself is a process that requires planning and resources that extend beyond completion of scholarly work. Mentorship and teamwork are as important during dissemination as they were during the actual scholarly activity. Maintaining support from the team will help to ensure that dissemination will be achieved and to elevate its quality. Consortia or collaboratories that seek to bring together multiple scholarly teams and overcome physical and institutional boundaries could further benefit your dissemination efforts.

Funding the dissemination process should also be considered. If you plan to disseminate your work at a conference, costs for registration and travel along with resource needs for poster or other presentation materials should be budgeted for. Journals are increasingly requiring authors to pay fees for publication, typically when an article is being published open access. If you plan to create a customized venue for dissemination, such as a website, dissemination costs could be high if they include professional site development and maintenance.

The time that dissemination will take should be accounted for, in relation to the urgency with which you need to disseminate. Recognize that those venues with the longest shelf lives also tend to have the longest processes for vetting prior to publication. Manuscripts and textbooks often take years before their content is available whereas social media allows instantaneous dissemination.

Understanding the limits of the resources you can dedicate to dissemination will help you choose among the options. You might also decide to delay dissemination while you secure the resources you need to attain good-quality dissemination results. You might opt for a combination, where you disseminate a portion of your work now, with plans to disseminate more later.

9.9 Credit, Accountability, Ownership, and Accessibility

Traditional peer-reviewed venues for dissemination have well-established conventions for authorship driven by the International Committee of Medical Journal Editors (ICMJE) [27]. Authors typically receive academic credit for a scholarly work and are expected to be publicly accountable for what is being disseminated. Proposed guidelines for scholarship in social media endorse the authorship criteria of the ICMJE [20].

While we have been referring to what is being disseminated as "scholarship," those in the legal profession might refer to it as "intellectual property." Indeed, peer-reviewed manuscripts often require a transfer of copyright from authors to the journal as condition for publication. Journals are increasingly providing options for open-access publications, which is a requirement for some scholarship generated by publicly funded sources and paid for by grants.

If you are disseminating resources independently online, then you need to be aware of whether you are sharing copyrighted material. For example, you would not be allowed to disseminate the complete text of most peer-reviewed manuscripts publicly online or through social media without permission from the publisher. The same would hold for videos or any other widely disseminated reusable learning object or online curriculum. Online, it is best to use material that has a Creative Commons license [28] or to refer others to the original source of a publisher and provide proper citation. When in doubt, seek advice from others, such as an online instructional designer, librarian, legal professional, or the appropriate office, policies, and resources provided by one's academic institution.

Ensuring that individuals with hearing or visual impairment can access your work will help it reach a broader audience and is considered a best practice in education [29]. It can be required by laws, such as the Americans with Disabilities Act

(ADA) [30]. Professional publishers typically manage these accessibility requirements for scholars, but if you are disseminating on your own, you should ensure that you comply with accessibility regulations. While laws are less prescriptive about accessibility to those with limited access to specific devices or the internet, considering how any online materials might be made interoperable on a variety of devices and software and accessible offline could make your work available to a broader audience. Again, if you are part of an academic or other large institution, it may be possible to consult policies or access resources provided by your institution.

9.10 Estimating Your Work's Reach

Considering that the influence of dissemination can occur over many generations as well as immediately, and that how we disseminate scholarship is changing rapidly, it is not an easy task to decide how best to measure success in dissemination. Indeed, there is no consensus in general on what measures best reflect the impact of scholarly work [31–33]. Traditional measures are still commonly used, but the academic community is becoming increasingly open to scholars providing the evidence that best reflects their ability to influence change.

Measures based on citations of a work of scholarship by another work of scholarship currently remain the most frequently used in health professions fields. Such measures make intuitive sense given that the purpose of dissemination is for scholars to build on each other's work to advance research and practice. Popular, single-number metrics include a journal's "Impact Factor" and "Eigenfactor" and an author's h-index.

Journal metrics are frequently thought of as a way to indicate the importance of a publication in correlation with a journal's reputation and number of readers. A journal's Impact Factor is calculated as the number of citations to all citable items published in that journal over a period of years, divided by the number of citable items published over the same timeframe. While the Impact Factor remains popular in some fields, some major professional organizations, such as the American Society for Microbiology, have eliminated it from journals under their aegis [34] due to concern that journals may compete for higher impact factors while compromising their obligation to disseminating the highest quality science. The Eigenfactor [35] was developed as an alternative measure that uses network analysis to weight citations based on the journal they are published in, thereby giving more weight to journals that publish more articles or are more highly ranked journals. The Eigenfactor also excludes self-citations.

The most commonly used citation-based measure for authors is their h-index ("h" coming from the last name of Jorge Hirsch, who proposed the measure). The h-index denotes the number of articles (n) authored by an individual that has n or more citations. For instance, an h-index of 10 means that among all publications by one author, 10 of these publications have received at least 10 citations each.

Limitations of these citation-based measures are well known, including variation that comes from different indexing sources (e.g., Google Scholar's is systemically higher than Elsevier's Scopus), wide variation across fields and disciplines, and incomplete ability to account for impact over time. Moreover, one cannot ignore the fact that these measures often reward scholarly activity where there is a high level of productivity among scholars while penalizing truly original works of scholarship in areas where few people are active. Finally, citation-based metrics may not reflect the methodological rigor or value to society of the scholarship [31].

Measures that take sources of data other than citations into account are gradually receiving greater attention. Altmetric [36] is a proprietary algorithm that seeks to measure the attention that a publication receives. It combines data from an evolving collection of sources that include social media platforms and web pages. Some have also suggested standardized methods of recording scholarly impact through social media in traditional academic CVs [37]; measures include number of followers and reactions to social media contributions.

There is also growing interest in going beyond quantitative metrics and contextualizing scholarly contributions in portfolios [38], through narrative impact stories [32] or through collaboration-based forms of evaluation of a scholar's contributions to the research community [39].

While the options for measuring reach described above are some of the more common approaches, this is a rapidly evolving area. As you consider how best to measure your dissemination's effects, it may help to consider its original purpose—for your work to be seen and appreciated by others so that they can apply it to their practice and scholarship. You can be creative in selecting what evidence you feel demonstrates how you have contributed to that goal. You can even turn measurement of your reach into its own scholarly project.

9.11 Conclusion

The impact of your work can be enhanced by how you approach dissemination. Knowing what and how to disseminate will help you decide which of the many options you could apply to your work. Ultimately, the service you can provide to the education and research community can guide the choices that you make and optimize your contributions in the near and long-term future.

Key Messages
- Effective dissemination connects your work with the people who can provide feedback and build on it.
- Many different types of scholarly educational products can be disseminated.
- Different venues for dissemination have respective advantages and disadvantages—focus on those that will reach the audience you want in the way that you want within available resources.

- Dissemination venues can complement each other; using multiple venues can improve the quality of your work and amplify it.
- When you choose your approach to dissemination, pay attention to conventions, guidelines, and rules of the selected venue.
- Dissemination itself is a process that requires planning, time, and resources.
- Dissemination makes your work public, so be mindful of intellectual property and accessibility issues and how you may be perceived professionally.
- Estimating the reach of your dissemination can help you appreciate the impact of your work and further inform your approach to dissemination.

9.12 Questions

Discussion Questions
1. What dissemination venues would you target for future dissemination of your work? What do you see as the trade-offs between the different options? (See Table 9.2)
2. Would you consider submitting your work to a preprint repository? Why or why not?
3. What in your view is/are the most appropriate measure/s to determine if dissemination has been successful?

Activities
1. Review the "Guidelines for Authors" for a journal that you consider a target for your scholarly project or instructions for submitting an abstract to an upcoming conference you will attend.

References

1. Merriam-Webster Dictionary. Disseminate. https://www.merriam-webster.com/dictionary/disseminate.
2. Cleland JA, Jamieson S, Kusurkar RA, Ramani S, Wilkinson TJ, van Schalkwyk S. Redefining scholarship for health professions education: AMEE Guide no. 142. Med Teach. 2021;43(7):824–38. https://doi.org/10.1080/0142159X.2021.1900555.
3. O'Brien BC, Irby DM, Durning SJ, Hamstra SJ, Hu WCY, Gruppen LD, Varpio L. Boyer and beyond: an interview study of health professions education scholarship units in the United States and a synthetic framework for scholarship at the unit level. Acad Med. 2019;94(6):893–901. https://doi.org/10.1097/ACM.0000000000002625.
4. Kern DE, Tackett SA. Dissemination. In: Thomas PA, Hughes MT, Chen BY, Tackett SA, Kern DE, editors. Curriculum development for medical education: a six-step approach. 4th ed. Baltimore: JHU Press; 2022.
5. Belton I, MacDonald A, Wright G, Hamlin I. Improving the practical application of the Delphi method in group-based judgment: a six-step prescription for a well-founded and defensible process. Technol Forecast Soc Chang. 2019;147:72–82. https://doi.org/10.1016/j.techfore.2019.07.002.

6. Wiley DA. The learning objects literature. Handb Res Educ Commun Technol. 2007;16:345–54.
7. Chen BY, Kern DE, Kearns RM, Thomas PA, Hughes MT, Tackett S. From modules to MOOCs: application of the six-step approach to online curriculum development for medical education. Acad Med. 2019;94(5):678–85. https://doi.org/10.1097/ACM.0000000000002580.
8. MedEdPortal. https://www.mededportal.org/.
9. MERLOT II. https://www.library.ucdavis.edu/database/merlot-ii-multimedia-educational-resources-learning-online-teaching/.
10. EQUATOR Network. https://www.equator-network.org/.
11. Norman G. Data dredging, salami-slicing, and other successful strategies to ensure rejection: 12 tips on how to not get your paper published. Adv Health Sci Educ. 2014;19(1):1–5. https://doi.org/10.1007/s10459-014-9494-8.
12. Varpio L, Driessen E, Maggio L, Lingard L, Winston K, Kulasegaram K, Nagler A, Cleland J, Schönrock-Adema J, Paradis E, Mørcke AM, Hu W, Hay M, Tolsgaard MG. Advice for authors from the editors of perspectives on medical education: getting your research published. Perspect Med Educ. 2018;7(6):343–7. https://doi.org/10.1007/s40037-018-0483-0.
13. Roberts LW, Coverdale J. Editorial decision making for academic medicine, 2021. Acad Med. 2021;96(1):1–4. https://doi.org/10.1097/ACM.0000000000003808.
14. Meyer HS, Durning SJ, Sklar DP, Maggio LA. Making the first cut: an analysis of academic medicine editors' reasons for not sending manuscripts out for external peer review. Acad Med. 2018;93(3):464–70. https://doi.org/10.1097/ACM.0000000000001860.
15. Mendes TB, Dawson J, Evenstein Sigalov S, Kleiman N, Hird K, Terenius O, Das D, Geres N, Azzam A. Wikipedia in health professional schools: from an opponent to an ally. Med Sci Educ. 2021;31(6):2209–16. https://doi.org/10.1007/s40670-021-01408-6.
16. Wikipedia. Criticism of Wikipedia. https://en.wikipedia.org/wiki/Criticism_of_Wikipedia.
17. Helming AG, Adler DS, Keltner C, Igelman AD, Woodworth GE. The content quality of YouTube videos for professional medical education: a systematic review. Acad Med. 2021;96(10):1484–93. https://doi.org/10.1097/ACM.0000000000004121.
18. Ting DK, Boreskie P, Luckett-Gatopoulos S, Gysel L, Lanktree MB, Chan TM. Quality appraisal and assurance techniques for free open access medical education (FOAM) resources: a rapid review. Semin Nephrol. 2020;40(3):309–19. https://doi.org/10.1016/j.semnephrol.2020.04.011.
19. Lu D, Ruan B, Lee M, Yilmaz Y, Chan TM. Good practices in harnessing social media for scholarly discourse, knowledge translation, and education. Perspect Med Educ. 2020;10(1):23–32. https://doi.org/10.1007/s40037-020-00613-0.
20. Sherbino J, Arora VM, Van Melle E, Rogers R, Frank JR, Holmboe ES. Criteria for social media-based scholarship in health professions education. Postgrad Med J. 2015;91(1080):551–5. https://doi.org/10.1136/postgradmedj-2015-133300.
21. KeyLIME Podcasts. https://keylimepodcast.libsyn.com/.
22. Must Reads in Medical Education. https://hopkinsbayviewinternalmedicine.org/must-reads/.
23. Fraser N, Momeni F, Mayr P, Peters I. The relationship between bioRxiv preprints, citations and altmetrics. Quant Sci Stud. 2020;1:618–38. https://doi.org/10.1162/qss_a_00043.
24. Maggio LA, Artino AR, Driessen EW. Preprints: facilitating early discovery, access, and feedback. Perspect Med Educ. 2018;7(5):287–9. https://doi.org/10.1007/s40037-018-0451-8.
25. Soderberg CK, Errington TM, Nosek BA. Credibility of preprints: an interdisciplinary survey of researchers. R Soc Open Sci. 2020;7(10):201520. https://doi.org/10.1098/rsos.201520.
26. DR-ED: An Electronic Discussion Group for Medical Educators. https://omerad.msu.edu/dr-ed-an-electronic-discussion-group-for-medical-educators.
27. International Committee of Medical Journal Editors. Defining the role of authors and contributors. http://www.icmje.org/recommendations/browse/roles-and-responsibilities/defining-the-role-of-authors-and-contributors.html.
28. Creative Commons Licenses. https://creativecommons.org/licenses/.
29. The UDL Guidelines. http://udlguidelines.cast.org/.

30. Burgstahler S. ADA compliance for online course design. Educause. 2017. https://er.educause. edu/articles/2017/1/ada-compliance-for-online-course-design.
31. Aksnes DW, Langfeldt L, Wouters P. Citations, citation indicators, and research quality: an overview of basic concepts and theories. SAGE Open. 2019;9(1):2158244019829575. https:// doi.org/10.1177/2158244019829575.
32. Friesen F, Baker LR, Ziegler C, Dionne A, Ng SL. Approaching impact meaningfully in medical education research. Acad Med. 2019;94(7):955–61. https://doi.org/10.1097/ ACM.0000000000002718.
33. Mingers J, Leydesdorff L. A review of theory and practice in scientometrics. Eur J Oper Res. 2015;246(1):1–19. https://doi.org/10.1016/j.ejor.2015.04.002.
34. Casadevall A, Bertuzzi S, Buchmeier MJ, Davis RJ, Drake H, Fang FC, Gilbert J, Goldman BM, Imperiale MJ, Matsumura P, McAdam AJ, Pasetti MF, Sandri-Goldin RM, Silhavy T, Rice L, Young JAH, Shenk T. ASM journals eliminate impact factor information from journal web-sites. Appl Environ Microbiol. 2016;82(18):5479–80. https://doi.org/10.1128/AEM.01986-16.
35. Eigenfactor. http://www.eigenfactor.org/about.php.
36. Altmetric. https://www.altmetric.com/.
37. Acquaviva KD, Mugele J, Abadilla N, Adamson T, Bernstein SL, Bhayani RK, Büchi AE, Burbage D, Carroll CL, Davis SP, Dhawan N, English K, Grier JT, Gurney MK, Hahn ES, Haq H, Huang B, Jain S, Jun J, Trudell AM. Documenting social media engagement as scholarship: a new model for assessing academic accomplishment for the health professions. J Med Internet Res. 2020;22(12):e25070. https://doi.org/10.2196/25070.
38. Cabrera D, Roy D, Chisolm MS. Social media scholarship and alternative metrics for aca-demic promotion and tenure. J Am Coll Radiol. 2018;15(1):135–41. https://doi.org/10.1016/j. jacr.2017.09.012.
39. Declaration on Research Assessment (DORA). https://sfdora.org/.

Chapter 10
Writing an Abstract

Emily L. Jones

10.1 Introduction

In the very early years of scientific journals, the consumers of information were primarily gentlemen scholars living through the Age of Enlightenment. Scientific advances of the Victorian era led to an explosion of related scientific discourse. Memberships in clubs such as the Royal Society of London swelled as did the number of and specialization of these scientific societies—some with the express purpose of publishing new journals or presenting papers in front of their memberships [1]. As more journals were published, it became more difficult for audiences to keep up with so much new scientific information.

This abundance of scholarship produced the need to be able to sort through information in an organized manner. The first scientific abstracts were not written by the author of the research but by writers hired to summarize research for busy men of science who did not have the time or more likely the inclination to go through every article being produced. In the early 1800s, the Royal Society used the word abstract to mean the summary—usually written by a secretary rather than the author—of a paper that had been read at a scientific meeting.

The advancement of science depends on the ability to publish research that is scholarly, well supported, methodical, and translatable to practice. With the number of publications on any given topic continuing to outpace an individual's ability to search or consume all content, the scientific community relies on the abstract. With its primary purpose to accurately communicate the contents of a manuscript without giving excessive detail, the abstract places the work in the context of scientific research that already exists, informing the reader whether the article connected to the abstract is relevant to their interests and merits the time investment to read.

E. L. Jones (✉)
Johns Hopkins University School of Education, Baltimore, MD, USA
e-mail: emjones@jhu.edu

A. S. Fitzgerald, G. Bosch (eds.), *Education Scholarship in Healthcare*,
https://doi.org/10.1007/978-3-031-38534-6_10

A well-written abstract that appropriately represents your work can pave the way to conference presentations and an article that is read more often, is cited more frequently, and is included in more reviews. Abstracts vary in length, usually with a maximum of a few hundred words, and they may go by other names such as executive summary or synopsis. They may be free form or tightly structured depending on the publication or the purpose they serve. Understanding how to craft an abstract that delivers maximum impact within the allowed word count is a skill that serves the health scholar over an entire career. In this chapter, you will learn why abstracts are important and how to craft a compelling yet brief abstract for your research paper.

10.2   Why Abstracts Are Important

The chief purpose of an abstract is to serve as a summary of a larger work. This simple statement is the key to an abstract's importance in general and why it is specifically important to an individual scholar.

Abstracts allow others to quickly scan research to determine relevance to their interests. This feature of an abstract is used in the reading of articles in journals, the visiting of posters at conferences, and the selection of articles for research. For anyone searching databases of literature, having concise and accurate summaries saves hours of work as opposed to reading through entire sections of articles to determine if the article is useful for their research. In addition, when searching databases for relevant and related research, often the abstract is available to everyone to read while the full text of an article might be held behind a paywall only for the subscribers of that database. The abstract serves to inform the database user which articles are worth purchasing.

For an individual scholar, an abstract is highly significant because it serves as the ambassador for the scholar's larger body of work. When submitting scholarly work to a conference for presentation, it is usually the abstract that is requested. Selection committees review the submitted abstracts, and based on the quality of an abstract, an offer to present either a poster or an oral presentation might be tendered. For a manuscript submission to a journal, an abstract is what is sent to potential peer reviewers asking them if they would be willing to perform a peer review of your work, and it is the abstract that will be the first part of the manuscript that they read when they perform the review. In both instances, it is the abstract that proceeds to make an impression of who you are as a scholar and what quality you have to offer from your larger body of work.

10.3   Writing an Abstract: General Guidelines

Most abstracts contain around 120–300 words depending on the journal or conference guidelines. Since space is limited, each word counts. Key or pivotal concepts should be included in the abstract, particularly those that are necessary for proper contextual framing of the abstract. If the manuscript is already written, it is okay and even encouraged to use the same language such as phrases or sentences in both the abstract and the manuscript. Doing so creates cohesion between the documents. It can be problematic to change the description of an issue between the abstract and manuscript as this can be confusing to the reader. For example, the phrase "student centered" and "learner centered" should not be considered interchangeable with one term being used in the manuscript and the other term being used in the abstract. Instead, a single phrase should be decided on by the authors and used consistently in both the abstract and manuscript. Consistency gives coherence between the two documents and ensures that readers do not get confused about author intent. Abstracts typically do not contain citations, so any assertion in your abstract needs to be backed up with evidence in the body of your research paper.

Abstracts are written in the past tense using the third-person point of view. The voice should be active rather than passive, e.g., "The authors reviewed the tests" rather than "The tests were reviewed by the authors." Any abbreviations used in the abstract need to be spelled out completely the first time they are used, even if they are spelled out in the manuscript since the abstract is a standalone document. The wording of the abstract should be free of jargon, kept simple, and not complicated unnecessarily. For example, the word "use" is often the word of choice over "utilize." When writing, it can help to vary sentence length and structure to avoid monotony and choppiness.

What to do
- Do write the abstract as a standalone document
- Do spell out acronyms the first time they are used in the abstract (and manuscript)
- Do ensure that the abstract and the manuscript match in major findings
- Do use the same phrasing in the abstract and manuscript

What to avoid [2]
- Do not omit key facts in the abstract that could give the wrong impression to a reader
- Do not include any information in the abstract that is not in the manuscript
- Do not use the abstract as an introduction to the manuscript
- Do not omit articles (a/an/the) to save on word count

10.4 Abstract Structure

Journal or conference guidelines will let you know how to structure your abstract. In some instances, such as for an essay, the abstract may have no formal structure. For research manuscripts, the structure often takes the form of Introduction, Methods, Results, and Discussion (IMRaD) though the section titles often go by different names. For example, the introduction section might be called "purpose" or "background." The discussion section might be called "conclusion" or there might be both a "conclusion" section and a "discussion" section. Even for an unstructured abstract, it might be beneficial to start with the IMRaD structure because it is such a logical framework. Ultimately, the most important thing is to check with the author instructions for your intended target submission platform and follow their guidance for the final format of the abstract product.

As a general guideline for allocating writing space, consider allotting
- Introduction—25% of the space to the purpose and importance of the research
- Methods—25% of the space to what you did
- Results—35% of the space on what you found
- Discussion—15% of their space discussing the implications of the research

10.4.1 Introduction/Purpose/Background

Lingard and Watling [3] suggest that one of the most necessary components of good writing is finding "a problem that readers will recognize and relate to." Once this occurs, the reader begins to feel interested in possible solutions and invested in the possible outcomes. Perhaps, it is a problem that they themselves are facing or attempting to solve with their own research. Maybe the problem you are working on will lay the foundation for a project they are considering. The best introductions to abstracts use this as an opportunity to identify the problem and contextualize how your research either addresses this problem or adds to what we know about the problem so that it might be solved in the future.

The opening lines of an abstract should contain the answer to three basic questions
- What is known?
- What is unknown?
- What is the question?

By answering these three questions, the introduction is identifying the problem contextualized in the existing literature and shows how your research either addresses a gap or adds to what we know about the problem (Table 10.1).

Table 10.1 Examples of problems with the introduction/purpose/background

Background: We developed a program combining online learning, independent work, and leadership coaching to address the leadership development needs of junior and mid-career faculty
Problem: There is no context to understand why this work is important or how it fits into the existing literature

Background: Leadership development using best practices supports the use of multiple delivery methods including on-site components, multiple sessions, and a longitudinal program. We developed a program to address the leadership development needs of junior and mid-career faculty
Problem: The background gives information about the literature and details about the program developed but does not give an understanding of how the research relates the two together or what the gap in the literature is

Background: Junior to mid-career medical faculty often move into administrative and leadership roles without formal leadership training. Many national leadership training programs target senior rather than junior faculty. We developed a program to address the leadership development needs of junior and mid-career faculty using best practices of multiple delivery methods
Goldilocks: This introduction is just right. It gives the reason for the program in the context of the existing literature and problem space, thereby exposing the current gap that the research is addressing in a concise manner

10.4.2 Method

This section of the abstract is where you tell your audience exactly what you did. Since abstracts are constrained to a limited word count, you will not need to describe every detail but will need to provide enough detail to allow the reader to evaluate the methodology. It should include study design and the who, where, when, and how.

Some key considerations that you will want to include are the study design including what was the protocol—whether the study was experimental or quasi-experimental, whether it was a random controlled trial (RCT), and whether the research was quantitative or qualitative or used a mixed-methods design. You should be clear about the study population, describing who exactly was included or excluded (age, race, gender, occupation). Where the study took place should be mentioned including the setting, city, state, and country. Follow the rule of writing out names rather than using abbreviations, even if it is commonly known to you, e.g., write out New York City rather than using the abbreviation NYC. Including the dates of the study is important, especially as time passes. The dates will help readers put the abstract in context for time and assist with relevancy. Dates should be fully written out to avoid confusion rather than abbreviated, e.g., write out Month DD, YYYY or DD Month YYYY rather than MM/DD/YYYY or DD/MM/YYYY. Describe the basic procedure of the methodology including the most important dependent variable and the main dependent variable and the method of measurement.

Key considerations to include are the following

- Study design—state the study design or protocol right away (survey, meta-analysis, prospective, retrospective, etc.), e.g., "The authors carried out a prospective survey …."
- Who—describe the study population, e.g., "… of 2nd-year medical students …."
- Where—include the setting, e.g., "… at an academic medical center in Baltimore, Maryland …."
- When—describe the timeframe including the year(s), e.g., "… between July 1, 20XX and Sept 30, 20XX."
- How—describe the basic procedure and most important independent variable, and then give the main dependent variable and method of measurement

The methodology of your study can be a secondary draw to your paper. If you correctly choose keywords to include information on your methodology, your paper will show up in searches for specific research methods as well as topic searches.

10.4.3 *Results*

The few sentences you take or adapt for your abstract results should concisely and specifically reveal the most important or interesting findings from your study. Abstracts are your paper in miniature form, but remember that their job is to summarize your work. This means that you will not include graphs, tables, equations, frameworks, or anything that supports these findings within your abstract. If your reader is interested in learning more about your results, they can read your paper which will include all the important data and empirical evidence to make your findings clear.

Key significant findings should be included. When working with a study population, the results of the selection process should be given. When working with percentages, include the raw number with percentages. Round percentages to the nearest whole number (50%) or one decimal place (50.0%), for example, 480 (50%) of the respondents; many respondents ($n = 480$, 50%); or 480 respondents (50%). Appropriate confidence intervals should be reported whenever possible, e.g., "[95% CI, #.##-#.##]." Standard deviations should be reported in parentheses, e.g., "mean (SD)" or "mean ± SD." When using p-values, report the actual p-values to two decimal places and state if it is statistically significant or not statistically significant, e.g., $p = 0.01$, unless $p < 0.01$ or rounding to two places would make a particular value insignificant. Do not round p values to 0 or 1. Instead, use $P < 0.001$ and $P > 0.99$, respectively. Secondary results are only included if they are important. Inferences, comments, and discussions should not be included, e.g., incorrect due to commentary: *"Our most important finding was …."* Instead, avoid commentary and stick to facts: *"X was significantly more Y ($p < .001$) after Z."*

10.4.4   Discussion Section

The Discussion section is where you need to explain the "so what?", explaining what the findings mean and how they fit in with the current understanding of the field. Those who consume scientific papers are not only interested in reading your work but also integrating it into their own. Leave room for others to do that. You are (hopefully) excited about your research, and your abstract can reflect some of that enthusiasm. Just remember that your job when writing an abstract is to describe and not defend your research. Descriptive methodology, ensuring replicability, should help in that regard. Having strong evidence will help as well.

What to do [4]
- Give a clear takeaway message telling the reader what the results mean
- Explain how the results contribute to the field and will change what they do
- Keep the discussion brief, in 2–3 sentences

What to avoid
- Do not make the error of claiming too much
- Do not speculate or force readers to make inferences
- Study limitations are usually not included unless it is necessary so as not to mislead the reader about the study's importance

Contextualizing your findings within the context of existing research helps entice the reader to be invested and interested in hearing more.

10.5   Authorship and Title

A standalone abstract should use the same authors and author order as the manuscript to which it accompanies. (See the chapter on manuscripts for a detailed description of qualifications for authors and author order.)

The title is an important part of the abstract and the manuscript. In fact, it is the single most important part of your abstract that will get it read and get your conference presentation attended [4]. To come up with a good title, start by considering the main message and keywords related to your work. Try variations of titles, putting the main message near the front of the title, and ask co-authors and other colleagues for their input on which one they would find most interesting if they were a reader. Keep titles short, and avoid abbreviations in the title.

10.6   Bringing It All Together

The abstract is a standalone document composed of the individual sections—Title, Authors, Introduction, Method, Results, and Discussion. Once each section is completed, it is a good idea to look through the sections again to make sure that the verb tense is correct. Even if you are working on the abstract while the research is ongoing, the abstract should be in third-person past tense. Now is also a good time to look for keywords that can help others find your work by increasing the likelihood that your paper will be returned by a search engine or database query. Consider including keywords specific to your project as well as the larger context of the domain in which you are working. Including keywords about your methodology and including the specific population or setting can also result in increased abstract viewing. Having a colleague or editor to assist with this process is helpful as they can provide a fresh set of eyes (Table 10.2).

Table 10.2 Sample abstract format and expected content

Expected content[a]	Example content[b]
Title should reflect the content and invoke interest	Title: LEAD: A leadership program for junior-mid-career faculty
All authors listed are qualified contributors	First author, next author, senior author
• Description of what is known about the topic • Identification of the gap in the literature • Statement of the research question that addresses a gap in the literature	**Background**: Junior to mid-career medical faculty often move into administrative and leadership roles without formal leadership training. Many national leadership training programs target senior rather than junior faculty. We developed a program to address the leadership development needs of junior and mid-career faculty using best practices of multiple delivery methods
• How the project was performed • Methods used to answer research question • Report on data collection and analysis	**Methods**: 79 junior-mid-career general internal medicine (GIM) faculty enrolled in five consecutive annual cohorts from 2014 to 2018. LEAD scholars participated in a full-day anchor session followed by selected workshops at a society annual meeting. They then participated in monthly online sessions, completed a project, interviewed a senior leader, and received leadership coaching from senior GIM faculty. The LEAD program was evaluated using Kirkpatrick's pyramid of program evaluation. Mid-program evaluation was performed for continuous program improvement. A five-cohort post-program alumni survey was sent to all LEAD alumni in September 2019 for program evaluation
Description of the data that answers the proposed question	**Results**: Respondents (RR 51%, 40/79) to the post-program evaluation indicated that the LEAD program was effective in helping participants understand what it means to be a good leader (93%, 37/40), become a more reflective leader (90%, 35/39), and apply principles of leadership to increase effectiveness in their roles (88%, 34/39)
• Clear statement of what the results mean • Discuss the findings in relation to what is known in the field • How can this information be useful	**Conclusions**: LEAD provides junior-mid-career medical faculty an opportunity to learn effective leadership skills and build a network. The LEAD program offers a program model for leadership training that is grounded in adult learning theory and can be offered with a flexible structure and at a low program cost
What terms make this information findable to others	Keywords: Leadership, faculty, education, networking, mentoring

[a]Adapted from Varpio et al. [5]
[b]Adapted from Fitzgerald et al. [6]

10.7 A Note About Keywords and Artificial Intelligence Software

It is wise to consider the impact of artificial intelligence (AI) software on searches and whether your abstract will get the recognition it deserves. Have you included keywords relevant to your topic? Many systematic reviews rely on machine intelligence to assist in screening at least the first round of abstracts for relevance to a particular topic. Tools such as Abstrackr and Covidence use artificial learning to sort through thousands of journal articles [7]. These tools are estimated to save between 9 and 67% of workload compared to traditionally conducted systematic reviews, depending on the size and complexity of the review [8]. This increased reliance on technology to screen abstracts means that it is more important than ever to be sure that you are using the words in your abstract wisely and with some precision as to the topic you discuss. You might want to consider keywords from adjacent topics that your paper may touch upon.

10.8 Conclusion

Spending time creating an accurate, concise, and strategic abstract can result in an increased likelihood of your work appearing in search results and, ultimately, citations. Your abstract should be a summary that is able to stand alone, meaning do not assume that someone has read or intends to read your paper. Even if it is not asked for by the journal, using the IMRaD format as a guide can help ensure that you have all of the necessary information included in your abstract. Positioning your research as the answer to a compelling research problem can increase the likelihood that your abstract gets read. Being sufficiently descriptive with your methodology can mean that your work will get read due to interest in your research methodology as well as your research topic. Having others review your abstract prior to submission will help ensure that the most read element of your paper will be an accurate and enticing way to draw others to your research.

10.9 Questions

Activities

1. Write the first two sections of a scientific abstract—Purpose and Method—for your proposed project. Include the following:

   (a) Title
   (b) Authors

(c) Purpose—background, rationale, question
(d) Method—design, major elements, main endpoint/tool

2. Use the abstract review template to check your work:

Abstract Review Template

Component	Prompt	Impression		Comments
		Yes	No	
Abstract Title				
	Circle Title Type: Descriptive–Interrogative–Affirmative			
	Title is clear, informative, and represents the content?	☐	☐	
	Title is catchy—not dull or too highly technical	☐	☐	
	Title is brief (<15 words)	☐	☐	
	Title is without abbreviation unless internationally it is an internationally recognized abbreviation, e.g., HIV, AIDS, or similar	☐	☐	
	Authors are appropriately listed	☐	☐	
Purpose Section				
	The length is appropriate (approximately 50 words)	☐	☐	
	Background justification is given (what is known)	☐	☐	
	Study rationale is explained (what is unknown)	☐	☐	
	Question to be answered is stated (what is the question)	☐	☐	
Methods Section				
	Length is appropriate (approximately 100 words)	☐	☐	
	The study design is clearly stated right away	☐	☐	
	The study answers the following:			
	Who	☐	☐	
	Where	☐	☐	
	When	☐	☐	
	How	☐	☐	
	The endpoint and tools used to measure them are described	☐	☐	
Writing Style				
	Does the writer use short sentences with varied structure?	☐	☐	
	Is the verb tense accurate throughout—past tense third person, e.g., "The authors developed a curriculum."	☐	☐	
	Is the writing free of unfamiliar abbreviations?	☐	☐	
	Is it free of jargon and unnecessary formal words, e.g., "utilize" instead of "use"?	☐	☐	
	Is the text well written and easy to follow?	☐	☐	
Summary Comments				

References

1. Kronick DA. Medical "publishing societies" in eighteenth-century Britain. Bull Med Libr Assoc. 1994;82(3):277–82.
2. Farmakadis A, Bradford A, DeVilbiss MB, Campi J, et al. Handbook for Academic Medicine Writing Workshop. https://journals.lww.com/academicmedicine/pages/informationforauthors.aspx.
3. Lingard L, Watling C. Story, not study: 30 brief lessons to inspire health researchers as writers. 1st ed. Cham: Springer International Publishing; 2021.
4. Cook D, Bordage G. Twelve tips on writing abstracts and titles: how to get people to use and cite your work. Med Teach. 2016;38(11):1100–4. https://doi.org/10.1080/0142159X.2016.1181732.
5. Varpio L, Amiel J, Richards BF. Writing competitive research conference abstracts: AMEE Guide no. 108. Med Teach. 2016;38(9):863–71. https://doi.org/10.1080/0142159X.2016.1211258.
6. Fitzgerald AS, Fang M, Lee RS, Gann J, Burnet DL. The ACLGIM LEAD program: a leadership program for junior-mid-career faculty. J Gen Intern Med. 2021;36(8):2443–7.
7. Harrison H, Griffin SJ, Kuhn I, Usher-Smith JA. Software tools to support title and abstract screening for systematic reviews in healthcare: an evaluation. BMC Med Res Methodol. 2020;20(1):1–12.
8. Rathbone J, Hoffmann T, Glasziou P. Faster title and abstract screening? Evaluating Abstrackr, a semi-automated online screening program for systematic reviewers. Syst Rev. 2015;4:80.

Chapter 11
Academic Poster Design

Daphne H. Knicely

11.1 Introduction

An academic poster—simply called a "poster" in the academic setting—is a way for health scholars to disseminate information about their work at conferences and scientific meetings. Posters are a concise manner of communicating key information in a visually appealing way. They ideally act as a conversation starter to discuss research in a more detailed manner. Therefore, the goal of the poster is to engage conference attendees and generate interest in the scholarship endeavor [1].

Health scholars often realize the importance of the poster presentations to communicate the progress of their research, to receive feedback from conference attendees, and as a bullet point on their curriculum vitae (CV). However, they might not realize the additional benefits of a poster presentation, including [2–4]:

- Creating a visual record of the research
- An alternative to a traditional conference presentation
- An entry point for the development of a presentation
- A catalyst for a manuscript
- Visibility and opportunity to network (which can lead to future collaborations, invitations for guest lectures, and offers to be on committees)

Conference attendees also benefit from viewing posters and hearing poster presentations [4]. Attending poster sessions at meetings/conferences allows the opportunity to see the work of others and offers the opportunity to:

- Learn about new research in the field

D. H. Knicely (✉)
Division of Nephrology, Department of Medicine, University of Virginia School of Medicine, Charlottesville, VA, USA
e-mail: DH3RA@uvahealth.org

© The Author(s), under exclusive license to Springer Nature Switzerland AG 2023

A. S. Fitzgerald, G. Bosch (eds.), *Education Scholarship in Healthcare*, https://doi.org/10.1007/978-3-031-38534-6_11

- Interact with other scholars
- Ask clarifying questions about ongoing research
- Develop ideas for future research

Depending on the conference or meeting venue, the poster requirements are usually given to the attendee and may include displaying the poster by either printed or digital format.

11.2 Poster Submission: Selecting a Venue

Many institutions of higher learning or healthcare organizations hold a "poster" or "research" day, or they might have an internal conference that includes posters to allow health scholars to communicate the results of projects or to promote best practices. These sessions at your home institution are often a good place to first present a poster. The audience is (hopefully) friendly, and the feedback you receive at this venue can then be incorporated when taking your poster to other venues.

There are also regional, national, and international conferences that allow for poster presentations. Some organizations offer both a regional meeting and then a national meeting or both a national and then an international meeting. If this is the case, it is a good idea to take the poster to the smaller venue first to get feedback and practice. You will then be better prepared when you take your poster to the larger venue.

There are factors to consider when selecting a conference for your scholarly work [5, 6]:

1. Conference focus
2. Opportunities to present your scholarly work
3. Networking opportunities
4. Conference and travel cost

In the audience, you might find researchers, academics, students, and/or professionals who want to keep up to date with the latest research. Some of those in attendance might be looking for potential research collaborators. Once you have selected a conference, health scholars should consider submitting their research for presentation.

11.2.1 Poster Submission: Via Abstract

The submission to a conference or scientific meeting is usually in the form of an abstract, and the poster is accepted (or rejected) based on its quality. An abstract is a summary of the scholarly work that explains the main points and is limited by a specified word count. An abstract can be *structured* (with subheadings) or *unstructured* (without subheadings). Submission guidelines specifying when abstracts are due, how to submit them, maximum word length, and whether/how to structure the abstract are usually posted on the conference/meeting website. If the guidelines do not specify if a structured abstract is required, then it is often best to use the more formal structured version.

Sometimes, the conference/meeting submission form asks if you would like to be considered for "presentation" if selected. When submitting an abstract to a poster session, being selected for presentation format rather than poster format is considered a prestigious offer. The honor is usually reserved for a select few who are deemed to be the very top submissions as determined by the conference or scientific meeting's selection committee based on a competitive review process of the poster abstracts submitted. It is recommended that a scholar say "yes" to this option if possible. It is a chance to gain visibility by presenting your research to a larger audience. When this happens, instead of creating a poster, you will be asked to instead give a formal (e.g., PowerPoint) presentation in an auditorium setting.

The abstract itself is not included on the actual poster but instead used as the starting point for developing the contents of the poster if accepted. However, conferences or scientific meetings will often display the accepted abstracts in a conference or meeting booklet or as a post on their website page. Before the poster session occurs, the list of abstracts as a booklet or website page acts as a program guide for the attendees to help them decide which research projects sound compelling. That way, attendees can plan their time and decide what posters to prioritize visiting during poster sessions. After the meeting, the abstracts act as a lasting record of the poster session and are often a citable research source.

11.3 Designing a Poster

There are different designs for a poster depending on your type of scholarly work. Some conferences will give you guidance for poster presentations, but sometimes this guidance might be limited. Guidelines might include poster size limits, poster orientation (landscape vs. portrait), required sections, word count limitations, font selection, or font size. If you are given guidelines, then familiarize yourself with them and follow them closely. Failure to adhere to these guidelines might lead to your scholarly work not being accepted [7].

Some institutions have preset poster templates. These are usually on a single PowerPoint slide that is editable. The detail on the preset templates might take the form of a color scheme and your institutional logo or might be as detailed as the exact location for the sections of information such as data tables and conclusions. Checking with your institution and division before starting your poster design is recommended.

If your institution does not offer a template, you can either download one from an online source—many print stores offer free poster templates—or start your own template using a PowerPoint slide. To make a template on PowerPoint, use a "Title

Slide" setting with a plain background in normal view. Because conference poster size can vary, it is important to set the aspect ratio for the slide. In PowerPoint, under the "design" tab, "slide size" is a drop-down menu. This is where adjustments can be made to the length-to-width ratio, so the full-size poster is correctly proportioned. It is a good idea to make this adjustment at the beginning of the design process because landscape posters with a width:length ratio of 3:4 are significantly different from ones that are 5:7. You do not want to have to make last-minute adjustments due to incorrect ratios. Once a template is made, it can be saved and reused for future poster presentations.

Start the process of thinking through your poster by considering what images you might want to include such as diagrams, tables, graphs, and/or figures. You want to keep in mind that there should be a balance of positive space (e.g., text and images) and negative space (empty or white). Not having enough negative space can make a poster less appealing. It is recommended that you keep the following design guidelines in mind [8]:

- 30–40%—negative (negative/white space)
- 40–50%—images (diagrams, tables, graphs, figures)
- 20–25%—text

The most important aspect of your poster presentation is the key message or finding you want to convey. The main purpose and key message should be easy to comprehend. Health scholars should provide only vital and essential information. There is limited space, so unnecessary details should be eliminated. When writing the text, use vocabulary that attendees will understand easily, and whenever possible, use bulleted short sentences or phrases rather than complete sentences.

It is often helpful to expect to revise your poster once you have gathered the component pieces together. Consider whether there is any redundancy that can be removed and if there is any visual simplification that can be done. Leave room for creativity in the way a message is delivered. Simple creative messaging can be impactful and memorable.

11.3.1 Formatting, Layout, and Color

A general rule is that the poster should be readable from about 3–4 feet away. This rule should help guide you on the font style and size that you use.

Font style: *Serif* is a font that has a decorative stroke that finishes off the end of its letters. Examples of serif fonts are Times New Roman and Cambria. Serif font can help with eye tracking while reading printed materials but can also appear cluttered and difficult to read. *Sans-Serif* or non-Serif is a font that lacks the decorative stroke at the end of the letters. Examples of Sans-Serif are Arial, Courier, Verdana, and Helvetica. It is considered overall easier to read. It is important to realize that members of the viewing audience are likely to have information processing issues at the same rate as the general population, so your design needs to make accommodations for the reading experience of these viewers. Such a design will benefit all viewers by optimizing the overall poster readability. In Yoliando's [9] comparative study of dyslexia guidelines, the following recommendations for font emerged:

- Font should be Sans-Serif
- The heading font should be larger than the regular text
- Avoid title case, capitalizations, and small capitalizations
- Use only Roman font (not Gothic lettering or italics)

Font size: The title font size should be at least 32, and the main text font size should be at least 18 [10]. Any labels or text for diagrams, graphs, figures, and references can be smaller but no less than 12. Exact font sizes are sometimes specified in conference guidelines, but if not, match the amount of information to the space while making the poster visually appealing.

Bold/Italics: Bold font is sometimes used for the title, section headings, and subheadings. Other text is not typically in bold font unless it is a single key point or concept within the main body requiring emphasis. It is suggested that health scholars **not** use a combination of bold with italics or underlining as this does not improve emphasis and can lead to a cluttered look and is difficult for those who have reading disabilities.

Alignment: Text should be aligned in accordance with the reading direction. For languages read from left to right, alignment should be to the left, non-justified. For languages read from right to left, alignment should be to the right. In general, the attendees or audience will read from top to bottom, so consider this when designing the poster and arrange the poster as vertical columns (not horizontal columns). It is also important to pay attention to detail and align your sections, keeping dimensions for diagrams, tables, graphs, and/or figures consistent. This is best done by using the editing view that includes a ruler and grid lines for the software being used to create the poster. White space along the margins of the poster should also be kept equidistant.

Yoliando's [9] comparative study guidelines for layout include the following:

- Text should be aligned but not justified as it leads to inconsistent word spacing
- Consider using bullet points and numbering
- Character spacing should be set to 0%; word spacing should be proportional
- Line spacing of 1.5 is preferable
- Abbreviation, hyphenation, and indentation are not recommended

Colors: A poster with color is more visually appealing than one in grayscale and will attract increased attention. However, it is important to design with the population who have vision deficiency in mind, 8% of males and 0.5% of females [11]. When using color, both color *contrast* (for readability) and *preference* are important to consider. Murch [12] found that effective color usage for readability involved basic principles including the following:

- Avoidance of the simultaneous display of highly saturated, spectral extreme colors.

Table 11.1 Color readability combinations [12]

Background Color	Better Background-Text Combinations	Less Favorable Combinations
White	Blue > Black > Red	Yellow > Cyan
Black	White > Yellow	**Blue** > Red > Magenta
Red	Yellow > White > Black	Magenta > Blue > Green > Cyan
Green	Black > Blue > Red	**Cyan** > Magenta > **Yellow**
Blue	White > Yellow > Cyan	Green > Red > Black
Cyan	Blue > Black > Red	**Green > Yellow > White**
Magenta	Black > White > Blue	Green > Red > Cyan
Yellow	Red > Blue > Black	White > Cyan

*Based on Murch, G.M., 1985, June. Colour graphics—blessing or ballyhoo? In *Computer Graphics Forum* (Vol. 4, No. 2, pp. 127-135). Oxford, UK: Blackwell Publishing Ltd.

- Older viewers require higher brightness levels to distinguish colors.
- Opponent colors go well together.
- Red and green are not well perceived with peripheral vision, so for large displays, use blue and yellow for symbols displayed on the periphery.
- Use color sparingly (Table 11.1)

Yoliando's [9] comparative study guidelines for colors include the following:

- Use less contrasted colors such as cream-black
- Use warm background colors (such as cream)
- Use matte finish rather than glossy finish to prevent light glare and reflection
- Cream and pastel colors are the easiest to be perceived for people with dyslexia
- Avoid backgrounds of cooler colors (blue/green)
- Avoid color combinations: yellow-black, white-blue, and combinations of grey

Awareness of the guidelines for color use will also ensure that your poster adheres to best practices of inclusiveness for visual and reading impairments. Consistency throughout the entire poster is important to achieve the highest level of readability for all viewers.

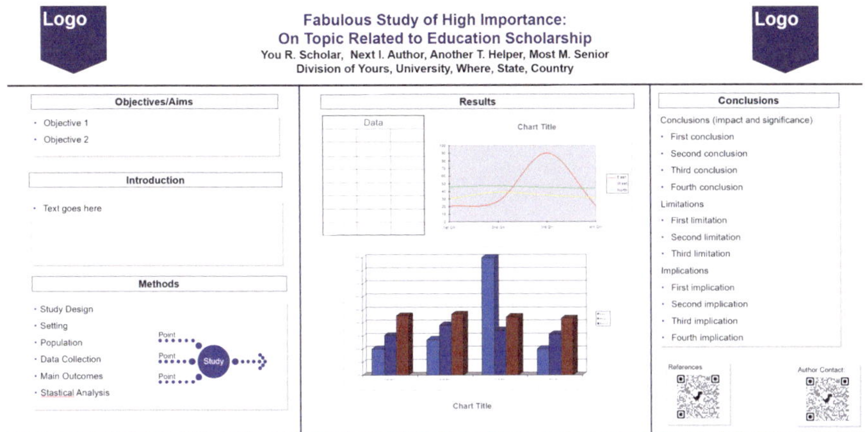

Fig. 11.1 Example of poster layout in landscape orientation

11.3.2 Poster Layout

The conference guidelines usually specify the orientation as landscape or portrait. The only difference between the two orientations comes in the formatting. Due to portrait's orientation, two columns of text are sometimes used. However, when considering readability, multiple columns are less desirable [9] (Figs. 11.1 and 11.2).

11.4 Poster Sections

The poster sections might vary depending on your specific scholarly work. A rule of thumb is about 100 words per section. Usually, the total word count for the poster (excluding banner, references, and any legends) should be in the range of 600–1000 words. Use diagrams, tables, graphs, and/or figures to explain a complex methodology or intricate data. This strategy will help to reduce the amount of text.

11.4.1 Banner Section

The banner runs across the poster's top margin. It occupies the top 20% of a landscape poster's banner and the top 15% of a portrait poster's banner. In this section is included the title, author(s), institutional affiliations, and logos/insignias for the institutions and/or funding source.

Title: The title is important to generate interest in conference attendees. It should be catchy but have a scholarly tone. Keep the title brief, less than ~15 words. The

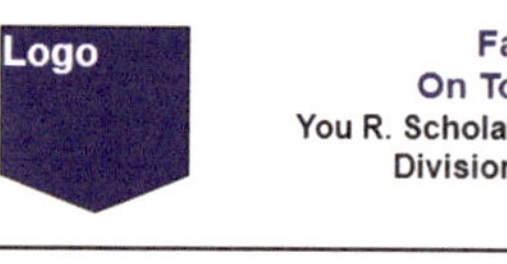

Fig. 11.2 Example of poster layout in portrait orientation

goal is an engaging and descriptive title that clearly conveys your research topic in concise terms without being overly technical or having extraneous details. Limit acronyms and generally spell out any that you use. Acronyms that are internationally recognized or widely known do not require spelling out, e.g., HIV, AIDS, and COVID.

Authors/Affiliation: Under the title, the author(s) names and institutional affiliations are listed in the same manner as they are for manuscripts. Institutions and/or funding organizations might also require their logos or insignias to be added to the poster.

11.4.2 *Study Design*

The first part of the poster explains the design of the study.

Aims/Objectives and Introduction: The Aims/Objectives section includes short statements that give the reader your project focus with clarity. They should indicate *what* your project is set out to achieve and *how*. This section should be bulleted. It is followed by (or sometimes combined with) the introduction. The introduction, also known as the background, explains why the scholarly work was created and sets the context for the project. Often, any background research is presented. It will list any gaps in the literature and what led to the research question and will justify the need to conduct the study.

Methods: The methods section is used to explain how the research was conducted. This section is used to describe details such as the population studied, setting, duration of the study, inclusion/exclusion criteria, recruitment procedure, study design, interventions, parameters studied, outcome measures, and statistical plan. Complex methodologies can also be assisted by a diagram or figure; this strategy saves on the wording.

11.4.3 *Study Outcomes*

The second half of the poster is the outcomes section. These sections describe the study data and help the viewer easily interpret the results and their meaning.

Tables: Tables are often used to show collected data. When designing a poster, it is sometimes tempting to put too much data in the tables section. If there is too much data, the viewers might suffer cognitive overload and miss the main message of the study. Keep this in mind and pare down displays to what is required to show evidence of your project's validity without being overwhelming.

Graphic Displays: Graphs and diagrams are helpful to simplify and transfer information regarding distributions, methodologies, concepts, structures, processes, and procedures. Creativity is encouraged to find simplified ways to convey your project information/results and to make it easily understandable for the conference attendee who might have little time to spend at your poster. General guidelines include the following:

- Your most important graphic should be prominently displayed
- The type of data determines the best graphic representation to convey it

- Any images should have a resolution of at least 300 dots per inch (dpi) to ensure print clarity

Conclusion: The conclusion section states the findings (impact and significance), limitations (or confounders), and implications (strengths) of the study. It should discuss any plans you have for further research or vision you have for where this study could potentially lead others in the future. This section is usually best expressed as bullet points. While "discussion" compares results from a scholarly work with earlier studies, the "discussion" and "conclusion" sections of a poster are often combined. The most important finding or "take-home point" should be easily recognized in this section.

11.4.4 Reference Section

The need to use references on a poster is variable as citing sources may or may not be necessary depending on how the poster is written and created. If citing a source is necessary, then references can be placed at the end of the poster or a QR code linking to them.

11.4.5 Contact Information

Posters are often presented at institutional meetings or professional societies where attendees usually have access to each other's contact through member registries. Still, it can be helpful to have the corresponding author's contact information labeled directly on the poster. This simple step can lower the barrier to networking or follow-up questions. Instead of the traditional mailing address, email, and/or telephone number, a QR code linking to social media can be used if the social media then also directs the user to more traditional forms of communication, e.g., a website link that then shows an email address or phone number.

11.4.6 Supplemental Information

QR (Quick Response) codes and the ubiquitous smartphone with a QR reader on its camera have made it simple to easily add supplemental information to posters. Contact information, references, or study information can be added to the poster easily with the machine-readable code consisting of a black-and-white square. QR codes can be generated by most computer browsers and then easily added to the right lower corner of the poster.

11.5 Digital Posters

Digital posters are also known as electronic posters or e-posters. A digital poster can be as simple as an electronic version of the paper poster displayed on a large monitor instead of printed on paper. This saves the presenter the cost and inconvenience of printing the poster and the hosting site the cost of the large display board. The interaction between the poster presenter and the attendees is otherwise the same.

However, the digital poster offers innovative forms of presenting health scholarship research [13]. Formats used for presenting posters in the virtual environment include the online gallery, asynchronous online sessions, and synchronous online sessions:

- An online gallery has posters hosted or stored online with online question-and-answer discussion boards for the poster
- An asynchronous session involves recording a video presentation explaining the poster. This type of session might include a live portion during the conference where attendees could question the poster's author.
- Synchronous sessions have the posters presented live online during a scheduled poster session and usually offer the opportunity for questions. Sometimes, these sessions involve going through sections of the poster as individual slides rather than displaying the entire poster as one slide. This approach facilitates clearer online viewing.

In any of these formats, the design and preparation of the poster board are essentially unchanged from that described in this chapter.

11.6 Finalizing and Presenting the Poster

Once the poster is finalized on the computer, it can be sent for printing. However, before that step, it is important to do a final check to ensure that there are no errors. A trusted colleague or mentor can help assist to do the final proof (Table 11.2).

Print options for posters include paper matte finish paper, glossy finish paper, or polyester fabric. Glossy paper is more difficult for those with a reading disability, so a matte finish is preferred to achieve better readability. Polyester fabric is an alternative option that is wrinkle resistant, fade resistant, tear resistant, and waterproof. The material can be folded and ironed, so it is also durable and convenient for travel. The cost is slightly higher than paper but can be a saving if the poster will be used more than once since the material will not get damaged while hanging on a presentation board or in transport between meetings.

Poster presentations are not all organized the same way, but usually, the presenter is required to put up (hang) the poster at a specified place and time in advance of the poster session. Often the window for hanging the poster is relatively short, especially if there are back-to-back poster sessions, so the board is in use by another

Table 11.2 Checklist for the academic poster

Double-check conference poster guidelines
Title is <15 words, catchy but scholarly, conveys the topic
Font: sans-serif text, no small capitalizations, avoid using italics
Layout: aligned but not justified, abbreviations minimized
Color: warm background, color used sparingly, matte finish
All sections and images align and are neat in appearance
No misspellings; Consistency in punctuation at the end of bullets
The main finding or key message is clear and easily visualized
All images have a labeled title
Margins are equidistant on all sides
A colleague or mentor has also checked the poster for errors

presenter just before your session. Ahead of time, it is helpful to ask how the poster will attach to the board—whether by pushpins, clips, or another mechanism. These are usually provided by the organization, but having extra on hand to secure the poster can be helpful in case they are needed. Poster presenters are given instructions by the meeting organizers for a specified time to be present at their posters. It is advisable to arrive early and plan to stay late to maximize networking and interaction with attendees.

11.7 Conclusion

Academic posters are a means of disseminating scholarly work. Their concise and visually appealing design attracts attendees at conferences and scientific meetings, enabling you to disseminate your research and network with potential colleagues. Poster formatting, layout, color scheme, and sections all play a role in advertising your scholarly work. Your academic poster will hopefully be a catalyst for future research, manuscripts, and collaborations.

11.8   Questions

Activities

1. Choose an academic society affiliated with your area of expertise where you might want to present your work:

   (a) Find out when their yearly meeting is held, what the timeline is, and the word count for the abstract:

   - (*Hint—you can Google the society's name + abstract, and a website with the answers might come up.*)

2. Most academic institutions or professional societies have a poster template for their members to use:

   (a) If you do not already have a copy of your institution's or society's template, ask around and find out where you can get a copy.
   (b) Once you have the template, keep it filed someplace easy to find in the future.

References

1. Gopal A, Redman M, Cox D, Foreman D, Elsey E, Fleming S. Academic poster design at a national conference: a need for standardised guidance? Clinical Teacher. 2017;14:360–4.
2. Barker E, Phillips V. Creating conference posters: structure, form and content. J Perioper Pract. 2021;31(7 & 8):296–9.
3. Bavdekar SB, Vyas S, Anand V. Creating posters for effective scientific communication. J Assoc Physicians India. 2017;65:82–8.
4. Durkin G. Promoting professional development through poster presentations. J Nurses Staff Dev. 2011;27:E1–3.
5. Gray B. Developing and writing a conference abstract. Int J Orthop Trauma Nurs. 2020;36:100721.
6. Lang R, Mintz M, Krentz HB, Gill MJ. An approach to conference selection and evaluation: advice to avoid "predatory" conferences. Scientometrics. 2019;118:687–98.
7. Berg J, Hicks R. Successful design and delivery of a professional poster. J Am Assoc Nurse Pract. 2017;29:461–9.
8. Baker D. Presentations: creating conference posters using PowerPoint. Oxford: University of Oxford/IT learning Program. 2012.
9. Yoliando FT. A comparative study of dyslexia style guides in improving readability for people with dyslexia. In: International conference of innovation in media and visual design (IMDES 2020). 2020. pp. 32–37.
10. Gundongan B, Koshy K, Kurar L, Whitehurst K. How to make an academic poster. Ann Med Surg. 2016;11:69–71.
11. https://www.colourblindawareness.org/colour-blindness/. Accessed 12 Apr 2022.
12. Murch, G.M., 1985. Colour graphics—blessing or ballyhoo?. In Computer graphics forum (4(2) pp. 127–135). Oxford: Blackwell Publishing Ltd.
13. Masters K, Treasure-Jones T, Elferink R. Teaching medical and health science students to develop e-posters with learning toolbox. MedEdPublish. 2018. pp. 1–14.

Chapter 12
Writing an Educational Manuscript

Michael S. Ryan

12.1 Introduction

Writing an educational manuscript for publication is a daunting but fulfilling task for health scholars. Similar to clinical, translational, or basic science research, writing educational manuscripts requires dedication to ensure a cohesive and grammatically correct narrative. A comprehensive description of how to write effectively for publication is beyond the scope of this chapter. Rather, the purpose of this chapter is to provide a starting point for the health scholar as they begin writing.

12.2 Authorship and Forming the Writing Team

Creating an authorship team is seemingly intuitive; it is those who are responsible for the work. But it can also be quite challenging. Do you include the statistician who provided consultation for the data analysis? What about the mentor you asked for input on study design? Or the colleague who provided high-level feedback before you submitted the manuscript? Once you have decided on the authors, what is the appropriate order? These questions are common challenges for junior and senior scholars. In the following sections, we address those questions by describing the qualifications for authorship as well as considerations for author order.

The best way to deal with authorship is to discuss this topic as early as possible, preferably before the study begins. In these discussions, the lead author(s) discuss

M. S. Ryan (✉)
Department of Pediatrics, University of Virginia School of Medicine, Charlottesville, VA, USA

Pediatric Hospital Medicine, University of Virginia School of Medicine, Charlottesville, VA, USA
e-mail: michael.ryan@virginia.edu

A. S. Fitzgerald, G. Bosch (eds.), *Education Scholarship in Healthcare*,
https://doi.org/10.1007/978-3-031-38534-6_12

expectations, assignments for writing (e.g., who writes which section), timeline, and authorship considerations.

12.2.1 Qualifications for Authorship

Fortunately for health professions educators, there is a set of established and generally accepted guidelines for authorship. The International Committee of Medical Journal Editors (ICMJE) [1, 2] provides four explicit criteria. In essence, the ICMJE qualifications state that a potential author must *substantially* contribute to a manuscript before it has been written (e.g., design, analysis, or interpretation), during the writing and/or editing (e.g., drafting or revising), and must approve the final product. The "and" and "or" in these sentences is critical. For example, one can qualify for authorship if they design the study OR interpret the results (i.e. they do not need to do both). However, they must also write OR edit the manuscript AND approve the final product. Many journals explicitly reference the ICMJE criteria in guidelines for authors, and some require formal attestation statements from all potential authors. For these reasons, it is valuable to consider the guidelines provided by this organization as the gold standard for authorship qualifications.

To help illustrate the criteria, consider three examples that frame the spectrum of authorship considerations:

- Example 1: A mentor meets weekly with the lead investigator to discuss the concept for a research idea. This mentor then conducts portions of the study and is tasked with writing the introduction section of the manuscript. This mentor reviews the final manuscript before submission.
- Example 2: A mentor meets once with the lead investigator to discuss the concept of a research idea. The mentor provides feedback, and this feedback is used to inform the final study design. The mentor does not directly participate in the research. The mentor is involved in conversations about the structure of the manuscript and provides input on the organization. However, the mentor does not draft any sections. Following the initial draft, the mentor provides a critical review including suggestions for modifying the structure of the methods section and the primary points raised in the discussion. The mentor reviews the final manuscript before submission.
- Example 3: A mentor meets once with the lead investigator to discuss the concept for a research idea. The mentor agrees with the plan provided by the investigator but makes a few suggestions to tweak the proposal. The mentor is not involved in the research but asks to review the manuscript before submission. The author provides feedback to the lead investigator after the manuscript has been drafted.

Examples 1 and 2 clearly meet the qualifications for authorship. While the mentor in Example 1 provided more significant contributions, both examples demonstrate significant contributions before the writing, during the writing, and during the final review. Example 3 is more questionable. In that example, one may argue that the mentor contributed to the design by providing feedback to the lead author.

However, the challenge is whether that involvement was *substantial*. Similarly, feedback that leads to a revision of the final manuscript may constitute critical revision, but it is much less convincing.

The mentor in Example 3 more likely fits the criteria for "acknowledgment" rather than authorship. Acknowledgments are formal recognition of contributions made to the manuscript that do not fit the explicit criteria of authorship. In most educational journals, acknowledgments are provided in written form on the manuscript itself. Importantly, these individuals must be notified that they will be acknowledged and must be provided a final version of the manuscript; however, their approval is not required for submission or publication.

12.2.2   Number of Authors

In general, anyone who qualified for authorship should be listed as an author. However, there are a few health professions education (HPE) journals that place a formal restriction, typically six, on the number of authors listed for publication. Additionally, many reference formats only permit a listing of six authors before the term "et al." is used. While the limitation on authors posed by journals may at times be appealed (e.g., multi-institutional study), it may be helpful to consider limiting the author number to manage the workload effectively and avoid the potential for difficult decisions and conversations after the paper is drafted.

12.2.3   Author Order

Though authorship considerations are at least reasonably straightforward, author order is a completely different animal. Put simply, there are no universal guidelines or standards for author order. In rare circumstances, journals provide guidance on author order. More commonly though, decisions over author order are dictated almost exclusively by convention and historical precedence.

In a recent study, Mavis and colleagues [3] surveyed medical educators to ask their perspectives on author order. Based on that study and existing literature, there are some general rules to consider:

1. *The first author* should be the individual who provides the most contribution to the study. If the project results from a student-initiated research project, that student should be listed first.
2. *All other authors* should be listed in descending order of contribution with one possible exception: it may be preferable to list a "senior author (i.e., mentor)" last. In considering placement of the senior author, it is worth clarifying up front that the designation of "senior" implies that the individual has provided mentorship on the manuscript. One should not place an author in the senior position based purely on seniority or experience.

Perspectives regarding the position of the senior author are inconsistent. Some feel that the senior author should be listed second if they made the second most contributions to the manuscript, while others favor placing that individual last. To determine which way to land, the author team should consider whether the journal explicitly provides guidance on author order and perhaps the promotion and tenure practices of participating institutions. Concerning the latter, some institutions specifically count the number of senior author publications, with the assumption that last-author position translates to a mentorship role on the manuscript. Therefore, in those cases, it may be advisable to place the mentor last even if they made more significant contributions to the manuscript than middle authors.

12.2.4 Workload Distribution

There are two general approaches to workload distribution. The most common practice involves a division of labor in which each author drafts a section(s) of the manuscript. An alternative practice involves the first author drafting the entirety of the manuscript and asking for a critical review from all authors following the first draft. The latter may be advantageous for a learner or junior educational researcher who wants to take a shot at drafting the entirety of a manuscript for the purpose of learning and feedback. In that case, the mentor (typically the senior author) often provides a first pass at review before sharing it with all other authors for comment. Any of these approaches is acceptable. Regardless of the approach, it is most important for discussions to take place in advance of writing and for the lead author to provide transparency regarding expectations for writing, authorship, and author order.

12.3 Target Journals

Journals vary widely in the types of manuscripts they accept, their format, and various other requirements. While it is possible to identify target journals after completing the manuscript, it can be more efficient to consider potential venues for publication in advance of writing. This can save time in the long run by ensuring appropriate formatting, length, and style.

12.3.1 Journals that Publish HPE Research

Broadly speaking, journals that publish HPE research may be lumped into two categories: dedicated HPE journals and specialty-based journals. Though there are several differences between the two, the most significant involves the readership.

HPE journals are read by HPE leaders (e.g., course directors, clerkship directors, program directors, dean's office members) while specialty-based journals are typically read by clinicians in the respective discipline. Both audiences have advantages and disadvantages.

A busy pediatrician may be less likely to read an educational journal than they are to read a journal in their specialty; thus, a publication in a prestigious HPE journal may never reach the private practice clinician to influence their practice. And the converse is true; an internal medicine clerkship director may never read the same manuscript if it were published in a pediatric specialty journal. For these reasons, it is advisable to consider a list of both HPE and specialty-based journals in a list of potential target journals.

Identifying target journals is challenging, but significant resources are available. For example, the Association of American Medical Colleges [4] provides and frequently updates an annotated bibliography of journals for educational scholarship. Similar options are commonly found on several university-based websites and may also offer consideration. Drafting an initial list is a helpful first step in determining where to send a manuscript.

Identifying specific journals in scope: Searchable lists such as those aforementioned provide a great list of potential journals. However, one needs to eventually narrow the list. There are several methods for narrowing a list to a more reasonable starting point.

Reviewing references: One strategy for selecting a fit for your manuscript involves reviewing your reference list. For example, let us say that your manuscript has 20 references. Of those, 10 are from Journal X, 5 are from Journal Y, and the other 5 are from several different journals. A strategy may be to target Journal X with your first submission. The reason for this is simple: if you have cited manuscripts in Journal X in your manuscript, your manuscript is likely within the scope of the journal. Therefore, it makes sense to target that journal.

Searchable database: Databases such as JANE (Journal/Author Name Estimator [2]), a Web-based platform, provides a list of suggested journals based on the manuscript's title, abstract, or keyword. By simply populating any of those items in a search field, the database provides a suggested list of journals, rank-ordered by "confidence" that the subject matter is a fit.

Other methods: It is also completely appropriate to use less formal methods to identify target journals. For example, you can ask a mentor or colleague for advice. Finally, a more time-consuming but still necessary method may be to dig deep into target journals to view their mission and scope. At times, you may also need to read some of their recent publications to get a sense of the fit for your study.

No conversation about journals is complete without the mention of predatory journals. This (un)affectionate term is used to describe a group of primarily open-access journals that offer the publication of manuscripts for a publication fee with or without peer review. Of note, not all open-access journals are predatory, and the requirement for fees does not necessarily indicate predatory status. Predatory journals are those which provide publication at a substantial cost, *without* reviewing the manuscript for quality. They often misrepresent their editorial board staff and use email spamming practices to solicit submissions under false pretenses. As a consequence, a publication in these journals may be dismissed by promotion and tenure committees. For these reasons, predatory journals are exploitative. Several lists of predatory journals have been maintained by individuals and organizations. It is valuable to identify predatory journals, and we strongly advise against disseminating work in these venues.

12.3.2 Understanding Article Types

In addition to considerations for journals, it is equally important to evaluate the types of manuscripts each journal publishes. HPE journals offer a seemingly infinite number of article types with each requiring some nuance to the structure, format, or contents. For example, *Academic Medicine* publishes six unique types of manuscripts and a seventh category called "special features." The manuscript types include a range of word count guidelines (<400 words for letters to the editor to <4000 words for research reports), formatting structures, and review criteria. This variability is common both within and across journals. Because of the sheer diversity, we offer two recommendations and a piece of reassurance.

Recommendation 1: Familiarize yourself with the article types used across HPE journals. You may even want to keep a table or list of the types of manuscripts, their frequency of publication, any specific deadlines for special issues, etc. Doing so will allow rapid identification of target journal(s) for each manuscript.

Recommendation 2: Carefully review the instructions for authors *before* you draft the manuscript. Failure to do so may result in an excellent manuscript that is far too long, short, or poorly suited for the target journal(s).

12.3.3 Targets (and Backups)

Once a list of potential journals and specific formats is identified, it may be intimidating to determine which journal to ultimately select. Do I aim for the "best" journal? A more realistic option? How do I know what is best or realistic?

First of all, there is no best journal. Journals have different missions and target audiences; therefore, what may be a great fit for one journal may be a terrible fit for another. Though there is no best, there *are* more and less competitive journals. It is therefore helpful to first familiarize yourself with various metrics that are commonly used to describe the relative competitiveness of journals. We then turn to methods for creating a list of potential target journals.

12.3.4 Metrics

The most traditional metric used to describe a journal's competitiveness or prestige is the *impact factor*. The impact factor is a numerical score that looks at the ratio of citations a journal receives compared to its total number of publications. Because higher scores mean more citations, it is implied that the work published in journals with greater impact factors has more impact on scientific or clinical practice. Though there are obvious challenges to this interpretation, higher impact factors correspond to more competitive journals. Therefore, the impact factor can serve as a useful barometer for judging the likelihood of acceptance.

It is important to recognize that HPE journals have a substantially lower "ceiling" for impact factor compared to general or specialty-based health professions journals. In 2021, for example, the highest impact factor of any clinical journal was the *New England Journal of Medicine* with an impact factor of 91.245. In contrast, the highest impact factor for any HPE journal was *Academic Medicine*, with an impact factor of 6.893. Generally speaking, highly competitive HPE journals are those with an impact factor >1–2.

More recently, alternative metrics ("altmetrics") [5] have been proposed to serve as adjuncts or replacements for impact factors. These metrics consider more modern measures of impact such as view counts, social media posts, and blog entries. Though these metrics are increasingly considered by promotions and tenure committees and may more accurately reflect the importance of work, the impact factor is still probably a better gauge of journal competitiveness.

12.3.5 Strategizing

In the ideal world, authors would identify the one journal that met all ideal requirements: right audience, optimal impact, and likely to accept. In some cases, this is exactly what happens. The author carefully targets an appropriate journal, and a positive result is the outcome. However, with decreasing acceptance rates and the extensive number of peer-review journals, it is increasingly difficult to make the right choice the first time around. Therefore, a strategic tiered approach may be required.

Figure 12.1 illustrates the tiered approach.

To understand the tiered approach, consider each journal on a spectrum that includes prestige (i.e. competitiveness) and fit. Some journals are a great fit but have less prestige, while others are high prestige but poor fit. A poor approach involves shooting for a high-prestige journal that is a content mismatch (e.g., Journal L). This approach is highly likely to result in rejection and is, therefore, a waste of time for

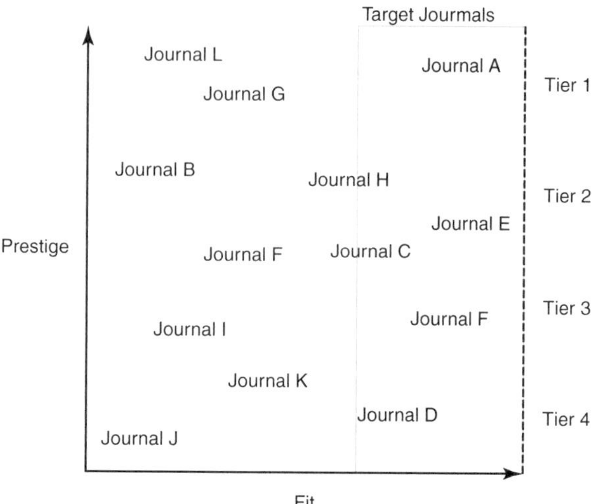

Fig. 12.1 The tiered approach

all parties. Simultaneously, it may be equally problematic to start by aiming for a low-prestige, high-fit journal on the first submission (e.g., Journal D). The latter approach is completely reasonable if one is concerned about time (e.g., promotion deadline); however, generally speaking, it runs the risk of underselling the importance of the work.

Thus, a tiered approach may be preferable. With a tiered approach, one begins by identifying a reasonable target journal or journals (e.g., Journal E or Journal F). Importantly though, these journals are *not* the first target for submission. Instead, one aims first for a "tier 1" journal (e.g., Journal A). For this first submission, the authors anticipate rejection but remain optimistic for either acceptance or at least a peer review. Even if the outcome is rejection, a thoughtful peer review may enable a more successful second submission, this time, to the more likely destination: "tier 2 or 3" journals (again, Journals E or F). If the second (or third) round of submission is unsuccessful, one also possesses a group of backups, or "tier 4" journal(s) (e.g., Journal D).

By working through tiers, the author assures the maximal impact and prestige of the journal while minimizing wasted time.

12.4 Writing the Manuscript

All manuscripts should follow one universal rule: maintain consistency and coherence between sections. A qualitative methodology should be informed by a research question that suggests that methodology. Discussion should follow from the results. The abstract should reflect the larger body of the manuscript.

Broadly speaking, educational manuscripts fit into one of four categories: research, innovation, perspective, or "other." In the next section, we distinguish between these types of manuscripts and provide suggestions for organizing writing based on the nuance required of each manuscript category.

12.4.1 Research Manuscripts

Research manuscripts follow a traditional format common across the sciences: Introduction, Methods, Results, and Discussion (a.k.a. "IMRaD"). This format is also pervasive in HPE journals and thus is the orientation worth considering for all research manuscripts.

12.4.1.1 Introduction

The introduction is designed to serve three goals: summarize the current state of the literature, identify existing gaps, and state the purpose of the current study. Easy enough, right?

The challenge with writing an introduction is that it is most susceptible to the "Goldilocks phenomenon." One must aim for a happy medium in which the background illustrates a sufficient understanding of the existing literature but not to the point of providing a systematic review. This balancing act is often hard to achieve, but there are two techniques to guide the writer.

Inverted triangle or funnel approach: This technique is the most commonly used in academic writing. With the inverted triangle, the author starts big and gradually narrows to the focus of the current manuscript. Starting big means identifying a healthcare level problem. A great example of this can be found in Starmer and colleagues' publication of the I-PASS handover curriculum [6]. From the first two sentences of the introduction:

> Preventable adverse events … are a major cause of death among Americans. Although some progress has been made … overall rates of errors remain extremely high.

In this example, the authors begin with a significant healthcare problem (preventable events leading to death). They then rapidly funnel the problem down from the healthcare system level to residency education—from residency education to curriculum development—and from curriculum development to evaluation of curricular effectiveness.

Most commonly, this approach uses separate paragraphs for each level of narrowing. A broad statement in the first is followed by incrementally more narrow paragraphs, concluding with a paragraph that explains the purpose of the present study.

Problem-gap-hook: Proposed by Lingard and Watling in their book *Story Not Study: 30 Brief Lessons to Inspire Health Researchers as Writers* [7], the problem-gap-hook (PGH) approach [7] takes a slightly different approach to the introduction. The authors argue that the readership of a journal is already interested in the topic, so it is not necessary to provide a comprehensive review of the literature. In their words, a manuscript is "joining a scholarly conversation," rather than *initiating* the conversation.

The PGH approach accomplishes a summary of the healthcare problem, articulation of a gap between current and ideal practices, and what is needed to close this gap (i.e., "hook"). All of this typically occurs within the first one to two paragraphs of the introduction (rather than across several paragraphs in the inverted triangle/funnel approach). The remainder of the introduction serves as an opportunity to expand upon those points in more detail.

To illustrate the difference between approaches, we can reconsider the I-PASS example. If the authors were to apply the PGH approach to the same manuscript, the following could serve as an outline of the first paragraph of the introduction.

1. Problem: "Preventable deaths may be linked to failures in communication, particularly during handovers."
2. Gap: "Despite ACGME requirements to provide handover training, the adequacy of training programs has not been rigorously evaluated."
3. Hook: "Effective handover curricula offer the potential to improve communication and thus reduce the incidence of preventable deaths."

Both the inverted triangle/funnel and PGH approaches conclude with a purpose statement, and typically a hypothesis. Most commonly, this is stated in the following manner: "… therefore, the purpose of this study was to … we hypothesized that …."

Theory, Theoretical Frameworks, Conceptual Frameworks

Regardless of the approach, it is critical to spend a segment of the introduction sharing key theories, theoretical frameworks, and/or conceptual frameworks that provided guidance to your work [8]. HPE journals are increasingly requiring an explicit statement of the theoretical and/or conceptual frameworks used to guide research in the introduction. Offering the lens for your work in this section sets the stage for methodologic choices, analyses, and discussion that follows in later sections.

12.4.1.2 Methods

The methods section should provide a clear and reproducible picture of what was done, to whom, why, and how the impact was measured. The reader should be able to, theoretically at least, replicate the study in their setting. This can be accomplished by continuously asking "why and how" questions. Why was the method chosen? How was this group of participants selected? Why were others excluded? Why was this method of analysis chosen? How was the analysis conducted? The methods section is also a critical component to the peer-review. The reviewer must understand the decisions you made in the design of the study AND agree with those decisions! Did you conduct an analysis using a statistical test designed for parametric data when the distribution favors a non-parametric test? Did you indicate a grounded theory approach but offer a design that is more consistent with phenomenology? For these reasons, we encourage consultation with an expert when writing this section, or better yet, to include them as a member of the author group from the onset of the study. A useful outline to organize the methods section is the following:

Overview. Provide a high-level summary of the methodology.

Was this a quantitative, or qualitative, or mixed methods study? What paradigm (e.g. constructivist, positivist, etc.) informed the study design? Was there a particular approach used? Why? Was it retrospective or prospective? Was this a single- or multi-institutional study? The purpose of summarizing the methodology is to provide a snapshot that serves to contextualize the rest of this section.

Setting. Describes in detail the environment in which the study took place.

The environment includes both the physical environment (e.g., "urban university setting") and the educational environment (e.g., "third-year pharmacy school curriculum"). The purpose of the setting is to establish the generalizability of the study. The reader should be able to determine "does this apply to my context?"

Subjects. Describes who was eligible and who was selected for participation.

What were the criteria for inclusion? Exclusion? How was this population identified (e.g., "we identified members of a listserv," or "all students at __ school were eligible")? Similar to the setting, the description of the subject helps the reader determine whether the study applies to their environment.

Specific method. A detailed description of exactly what happened in the study.

Most commonly, a chronological approach is ideal: "First we identified eligible participants … Next, we administered a pre-test … Then, we …." This allows the reader to follow along in the steps to determine if there was a logical approach.

Instrument(s). Description of measurements used to determine impact.

Similar to the previous section, this section should also be sufficiently detailed to include all important characteristics of the instruments. This includes, if applicable, the name(s) of the instrument(s) (e.g. Maslach Burnout Inventory), number of items, range of scores (e.g., "scale of 1–5 where 1 = __, 5 = __"), and any other factors that will allow the reader to determine how methods were operationalized. For instruments previously cited in the literature, citations should be provided. The instrument(s) should be provided either as a formal exhibit (i.e., table/figure) or as a supplemental file.

Analysis. The specific analytical approach that was used in the study.

For quantitative research, this should include the name of the statistical tests and significance values (e.g., "p-value of <0.05 was established for significance"). For qualitative research, the authors should describe the analytical approach in sufficient detail to allow replication and pair that with a reflexivity statement (perspective the authors/investigators brought to the study which influence interpretation).

Ethical approval. Statement of IRB approval or exemption

The methods section typically concludes with a statement regarding ethical approval.

12.4.1.3 Results

General Considerations

Consistent with the cardinal rule, the results section should flow logically from the methods. All measures introduced in the preceding section should be included in the results section, and in general, the order should be preserved. In other words, if two measures are introduced in the methods section, the results of those measures are illustrated in the same order in the results section.

The second most important consideration for this section relates to summarization. The narrative components should provide a high-level summary of what was found rather than a complete verbatim statement of the data. Simultaneously, the results should not veer into the interpretation. That is left to the discussion. For example, "participants in both groups were similar in terms of their demographic characteristics" is a good way to describe results, where male participants were 48% of the sample and female participants were 52%. The example maintains objectivity but still offers summarization to minimize the workload for the reader.

Organization

The results section typically begins with a summary of the participants and their characteristics. This is affectionately referred to as "table 1" data. Even if a formal table is not included, the first paragraph generally includes a summary of who participated and what groups they represent (e.g., demographic data). For quantitative studies, it is often advisable to describe who *did not* participate in the study. This may include a formal calculation of "response rate" or a descriptor of how many participants were excluded from the study and for what reasons (e.g., "10 participants were excluded … 5 did not complete the survey in its entirety and 5 did not provide demographic data for analysis).

The remainder of the section should provide a summary of the data, in a mixture of numerical, narrative, graphical, and tabular formats. Qualitative studies are typically summarized in a slightly different manner depending on the specific qualitative method used. Generally, most qualitative manuscripts are organized in such that paragraphs center on themes with summaries of those themes provided in table form. Exemplar quotes may be provided within the main text or in tables. Challenges involved in writing this section involve the sheer quantity and infinite options for displaying the data. A good rule of thumb is that figures and tables should be used sparingly and only when narrative text is unable to provide an adequate explanation.

12.4.1.4 Discussion

The discussion section offers the most flexibility but also the greatest opportunity for pitfalls. This section provides meaning and offers an interpretation. It translates the purpose of the study, offered in the introduction, and the findings described in objective form within the results into something the readers can take home and apply to their work.

So, how do we write a discussion? Because of the flexibility in this section, it is perhaps most beneficial to first share the constants: the beginning and end of the discussion.

The Beginning

The opening of the discussion commonly summarizes the purpose of the study, the major findings, and why these findings matter. Using this approach ensures that the author follows the cardinal rule and provides a clear and cohesive narrative to the reader. For many authors, this is accomplished through one brief initial paragraph in the discussion section. For example, "The purpose of this study was to … overall we found … these findings contribute significantly to our understanding of …."

The End

The final section of the discussion consists of two components: limitations and conclusions. The limitations section provides an opportunity for the author to reflect on potential issues with the study in terms of design choice, participants, etc. The reason for including this section is the view that reflective critique is an integral component of scholarly work. The purpose is to anticipate, acknowledge, and then rationalize potential threats to the validity of the study in a way that recognizes these limitations. However, authors should be cautious against sharing any limitation that may be viewed as a fatal flaw. By this point, it is too late to redesign the study!

The conclusions section provides one final opportunity to encapsulate the study for the reader. The specific format varies from a brief summary of what was found to implications for practice, next steps for research, or a "call to action," for the readership. Though this section should not deviate greatly from what was studied, this section provides the author with the ability to make a significant final statement: "… these results demonstrate a clear need for curricular reform …."

Everything Else

Now that we understand the beginning and end of the discussion, perhaps the middle feels a little less daunting. There are several key principles to consider when writing the "meat" of the discussion. First, all points raised in the discussion should relate to the study. It is appropriate to hypothesize based on the results or to offer a potential explanation, but it is not appropriate to tangent too far from the study outcomes. Second, ideas generated should be constantly compared to the existing literature and the conceptual or theoretical frameworks provided in the introduction. Offering a new theory is an excellent function of the discussion if it is indeed a *new* theory. Keep in mind that the manuscript is considered valuable, only if it fits a notable gap. Therefore, it is important to conduct a literature review to inform statements not just in the introduction but also in the discussion.

The specific method for formulating this section is a matter of style. Some authors will select a few "interesting" findings from the results, offer explanations/hypotheses, circle back to the original research question, and leave it there. Others will perform a more in-depth exploration of one particularly interesting finding. Still, others will use the results to offer a new theory or to expand or translate an existing theory to a new setting. This latter approach is particularly prevalent and valuable in qualitative studies.

Regardless of the specific style selected for the bulk of the discussion, it is important to spend time on this section. Lack of effort in formulating a thoughtful discussion raises questions about the practical or theoretical significance of the findings and questions about the contribution of the manuscript compared to the existing literature.

12.4.2 Innovation Manuscripts

The second common form of HPE manuscripts can be characterized broadly as innovation manuscripts. Though each respective journal has slightly different terminology (i.e., "innovation report," "educational innovations," "innovation"), the fundamental purpose of these manuscripts is similar: they offer the opportunity for educators to share the results of relatively novel ideas in HPE. Frequently, this type of manuscript is used to describe small-scale (e.g., one institution) studies that may or may not have robust results.

In general, innovation manuscripts roughly follow the same format as research manuscripts with two notable exceptions. First, these manuscripts tend to be shorter. Second, the terminology used for each section may be slightly different. This latter point is not universal. For example, the *Journal of Graduate Medical Education* uses the same modification of IMRaD for both research manuscripts and educational innovations (background, objective, methods, results, conclusions). In contrast, *Academic Medicine* requires a complete modification (introduction = problem, method = approach, results = outcomes, discussion = next steps).

Besides the formatting differences, there are several other important considerations for innovation-type manuscripts:

1. An innovation report should describe something innovative; it is in the title after all! The emphasis is on novelty rather than outcomes.
2. Though the focus is on innovation, this does not obviate the need for some results and critical reflection. For innovations, it is particularly important to highlight feasibility in terms of cost, time, or other resources.
3. Despite the novelty, the manuscript should still be important to the larger academic community.

The best way to illustrate effective innovation manuscripts is to consider an example:

Mary Andrews and colleagues successfully published an educational innovation in *Academic Medicine* on a novel approach to help internal medicine residents improve on their in-training examinations.

> *Andrews MA, Kelly WF, DeZee KJ. Why does this learner perform poorly on tests? Using self-regulated learning theory to diagnose the problem and implement solutions. Acad Med. 2018;93:612–615* [9].

The innovation described an important and generalizable problem in medical education (i.e., test-taking skills); it used a well-constructed theoretical framework to drive the intervention (self-regulated learning theory); the authors provided a complete and thorough description of the methods such that all readers could readily adopt the process; and the results demonstrated feasibility. The manuscript itself included multiple supplemental appendices including an open-access video that could be used by any interested faculty member. However, the study was conducted at one institution with a relatively small number of trainees. The outcomes were somewhat modest, but the intervention was feasible. For all of these reasons, this was a perfect fit for an innovation manuscript in a major HPE journal; but may have resulted in a less-desirable outcome if submitted as a research paper.

12.4.3   Perspectives

The third major category of HPE manuscripts is perspectives. Perspectives are *not* letters to the editor. The latter offers a direct rebuttal or viewpoint on a particular manuscript published within the respective journal. In contrast, a perspective is typically a commentary grounded in the literature and/or viewpoint of the author(s) and which is of direct relevance to the readership of the journal.

12.4.3.1   Why Journals Publish Perspectives

Journals publish perspectives for several reasons. First, perspectives offer an opportunity to discuss relevant topics that are either outside the realm of scientific inquiry or important to the readership but for which there have not yet been studies. A good example of this includes a series of perspectives centered around healthcare disparities and systemic racism following the George Floyd murder in 2020. The purpose of these perspectives was to call attention to an issue that was not yet addressed in the HPE literature.

The second reason journals publish perspectives may be somewhat surprising: these manuscript types are frequently the most cited manuscripts in major journals. Because of their provocative nature and timeliness, the perspective manuscript, more so than research manuscripts, creates a larger stir and formulates the basis for future scientific study.

And finally, perspectives are commonly *not included* in the denominator of impact factor calculations. Because these are not "articles" per se, their publication involves low risk and high reward.

12.4.3.2 Format

The format of perspective manuscripts is incredibly diverse and flexible. Few journals offer concrete guidelines for the structure outside of restrictions on word count. Because of this variety, we recommend that authors consider reading several perspective articles in HPE journals to get a sense of the flavor of what is accepted for publication in this category.

12.4.4 Other

Research, innovation, and perspective manuscripts are the most common article types accepted across HPE journals. However, there are countless other types as well. Some of these include shortened versions of the aforementioned manuscript types (i.e., "brief reports" or "short communications"), while others are distinct but highly journal-specific options (e.g., "validation" in *Teaching and Learning in Medicine, "foundations" in Journal of Continuing Education in the Health Professions*). Importantly, some of the manuscript types are only available in certain timeframes (e.g., quarterly), and therefore it is valuable for authors to review these potential venues on a case-by-case basis.

12.5 Additional Pearls for Success

As stated at the outset, this chapter is not a comprehensive guide to writing educational manuscripts. We hope that it serves as an introduction. In this final section, we describe a couple of important final considerations to optimize the chance for success.

12.5.1 Make Time

Health professions educators are busy. We often navigate between patient care activities, educational responsibilities, administration, and personal lives. Writing education scholarship is time consuming and can take a backseat if we are not careful. It is therefore important to carve out time for our writing.

We can make time to write by using several strategies. First, we can block off time on our calendars. The duration is likely variable for individuals. Some may prefer a large block of time (half-day), while others prefer to work in smaller chunks. Regardless of your preference, setting aside time is imperative. Second, we can maintain regular meetings with our writing team. It is often best to identify weekly meetings at the start of a project to maintain momentum and then back down slowly to less frequent meetings when the project is up and running. Maintaining this structure ensures that accountability is given to all members.

12.5.2 Invest in a Citation Manager

Citation managers allow for population of a reference list and automatic updates when changes are made. There are two reasons to invest in a citation/reference manager. First, it is nearly impossible to keep track of which citation is #23 vs. #24 following round after round of revisions. Inevitably, you will lose track of which was which. This can lead to frustration, or rarely, a journal may reject a manuscript outright if there are significant errors in formatting or numbering the references section. Second, journals use a variety of formats. If a manuscript is rejected from one journal, it can be massively time consuming to revise the entire format to meet the new journal requirements. With citation managers, this work takes about 5 s, following the simple click of the mouse. Multiple citation managers are available, some free, and some requiring a subscription cost. Most universities provide free or reduced access to a citation manager.

12.5.3 Consider an "Unofficial" Peer Review

The formal peer review (next chapter) occurs after the submission of the manuscript. But this does not mean that you need to wait until submission to obtain feedback. Identifying a group of colleagues who are willing to trade manuscripts for thoughtful critique is an invaluable way of gaining insight before the official peer review. This will allow you to make changes in advance of submission, thereby reducing (though not eliminating) the risk of rejection. When forming this group, it is important to identify individuals who may be willing to provide constructive critique. But you must also be willing to hear it!

12.5.4   Write a Cover Letter

Almost all journals offer authors the opportunity to write an "optional" cover letter. The cover letter is a note directly from the author to the editor. Because of this direct route to the editor, do not pass it up! In a succinct manner (~3 sentences), summarize what you did, what you found, and why this is of importance to the readership of the journal. Also, include any specific requirements the journal provides; most often, this is a statement about authorship and/or verification that the manuscript is not under review at another journal.

12.5.5   Double- or Triple-Check Your Work Before Submitting

Finally, it is extremely important to double- or triple-check work before clicking the submit button. Though small typos are likely to be tolerated, bigger errors may result in rejection or, at minimum, resubmission. One strategy we commonly use is the "sleep on it approach." Get everything ready to submit, but do not submit. Your work will be there waiting for you the next day. When you look the next morning, you will be ready to review more carefully than after a long day of finalizing the manuscript. It can be amazing how many errors you find after a good night's sleep!

12.6   Conclusion

Writing educational scholarship is a fun and rewarding process. With the possible exception of grants, peer-reviewed manuscripts remain the gold standard of promotion and tenure decisions at most universities. Becoming skilled at writing is a process that requires careful planning, formulation of a high-functioning team, and organization on the part of all authors. Once our work is complete, it is off to the peer-review process!

12.7   Questions

Discussion Questions
1. Type an abstract you have been working on into "JANE" (https://jane.biosemantics.org)

    (a) What journals came up in the search?
    (b) Are you surprised by what you found?

2. From a target journal of your choice, identify a journal format that is new to you.

    (a) What are the unique features of this manuscript type?
    (b) Do you have an idea that could fit into that description?

Activities
1. Create an authorship grid for a project you are working on. List the authors' names in order, and then detail their roles and responsibilities.
2. Create a tiered list of journals for the project you are working on. Identify at least one "reach" journal, two reasonable targets, and one backup.

References

1. International Committee of Medical Journal Editors. Defining the roles of authors and contributors. https://www.icmje.org/recommendations/browse/roles-and-responsibilities/defining-the-role-of-authors-and-contributors.html
2. JANE. https://jane.biosemantics.org/
3. Mavis B, Durning SJ, Uijtdehaage S. Authorship order in medical education publications: in search of practical guidance for the community. Teach Learn Med. 2019;31:288–97.
4. AAMC-Regional Groups on Educational Affairs (GEA): Annotated bibliography of journals for educational scholarship. 2022. https://www.aamc.org/media/38166/download
5. Meyer HS, Artino A, Maggio LA. Tracking the scholarly conversation in health professions education: an introduction to altmetrics. Acad Med. 2017;92:1501.
6. Starmer AJ, O'Toole JK, Rosenbluth G, et al. Development, implementation, and dissemination of the I-PASS handoff curriculum: a multisite educational intervention to improve patient handoffs. Acad Med. 2014;89:876–84.
7. Lingard L, Watling C. Story, not study: 30 brief lessons to inspire health researchers as writers. Springer International Publishing. 2021.
8. Varpio L, Paradis E, Uijtdehaage S, Young M. The distinctions between theory, theoretical framework, and conceptual framework. Acad Med. 2020;95:989–94.
9. Andrews MA, Kelly WF, DeZee KJ. Why does this learner perform poorly on tests? Using self-regulated learning theory to diagnose the problem and implement solutions. Acad Med. 2018;93:612–5.

Chapter 13
Peer Review

Michael S. Ryan

13.1 Introduction

Spier [1] described peer review as *"a turf battle with the ultimate prize of the knowledge, science or doctrine being published. On the one side, we have the writers and originators of ideas, on the other, we have the editors and critics."* Peers reviewing the work of a contemporary is a practice that dates to ancient Syria and Greece, but many historians attribute the beginning of modern peer review to England in the early 1700s. Before this time, publication contents were seen as the purview of an editor and possibly anyone he might have sought to assist him. It was the Royal Society of Edinburgh that started a process as early as 1731 that subjected manuscripts to a review procedure including inspection by a select group of individuals who were knowledgeable in the subject matter of the manuscript and whose recommendation to the editor would influence the future of the manuscript publication [1].

The purpose of the peer-review process is quality assurance. Peer review assures the integrity of the work. This assurance means that someone who knows what the original investigators were doing has double-checked the contents of the manuscript before it was published. Through careful selection of reviewers, the editorial board of a journal assures the readership that the work was conducted ethically with appropriate methods and analysis that led to a justified conclusion. Even if a reader is unfamiliar with the topic of a study, the reader should be able to trust the peer reviewer's judgment that the work meets standards of scientific quality. Peer review is about establishing and maintaining trust and credibility. Since science builds on science, trust is imperative.

M. S. Ryan (✉)
University of Virginia School of Medicine, Pediatric Hospital Medicine,
Charlottesville, VA, USA
e-mail: michael.ryan@virginia.edu

A. S. Fitzgerald, G. Bosch (eds.), *Education Scholarship in Healthcare*,
https://doi.org/10.1007/978-3-031-38534-6_13

Not only is peer review integral to scholarship, but it is also an essential component of an effort for it to qualify as scholarship.

- *Scholarly teaching* is defined as the process by which one defines a gap in the literature, identifies a research question, performs an intervention, obtains results, and analyzes the outcomes [2].
- *Scholarship* includes the criteria for scholarly work plus three additional steps that occur through dissemination. These are commonly referred to as the three **P**s—the work must be made **p**ublic, re**p**roducible by others, and subject to **p**eer review [3].

Even the most important, groundbreaking manuscripts could only be considered scholarly work without being subject to peer review (Fig. 13.1).

The peer-review process also has benefits for the author. While it can be difficult to invite others to critically appraise our work, constructive feedback is essential to the growth of any scholar. Many of us have experienced submitting a "perfect manuscript" only to receive peer feedback from a reviewer highlighting ideas for improvement and insights that we had not considered. The suggestions result in an improved final product and gratefulness for the peer-review process.

13.2   The Peer-Review Process

Now that we understand some of the reasons for peer review, let us consider the process itself. It is important to recognize up front that peer review is a method that requires adequate (lengthy) time to accomplish. In our experience, the time from initial submission to initial decision takes about 4 months. The time from initial submission to final decision takes about 6–9 months.

A helpful guide that is specific to Academic Medicine but may also apply to many other health professions education journals was developed by Durning and Carline [4]. Though each journal conducts its peer review in a slightly different way, there are general stages to which most journals adhere. Figure 13.2 provides a summary of these stages including a description, the responsible individual, and a typical timeframe.

Fig. 13.1 The relationship between scholarly work and scholarship

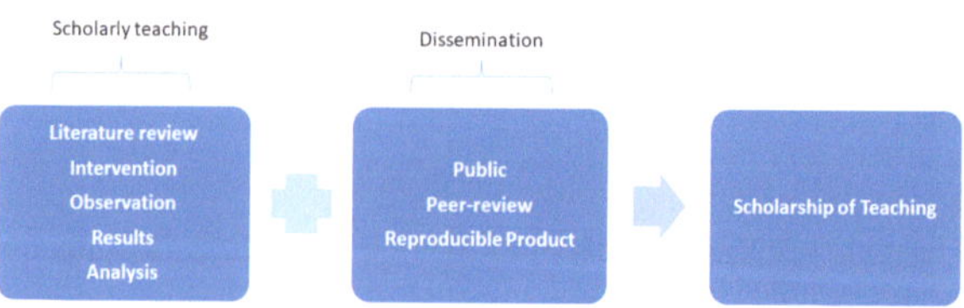

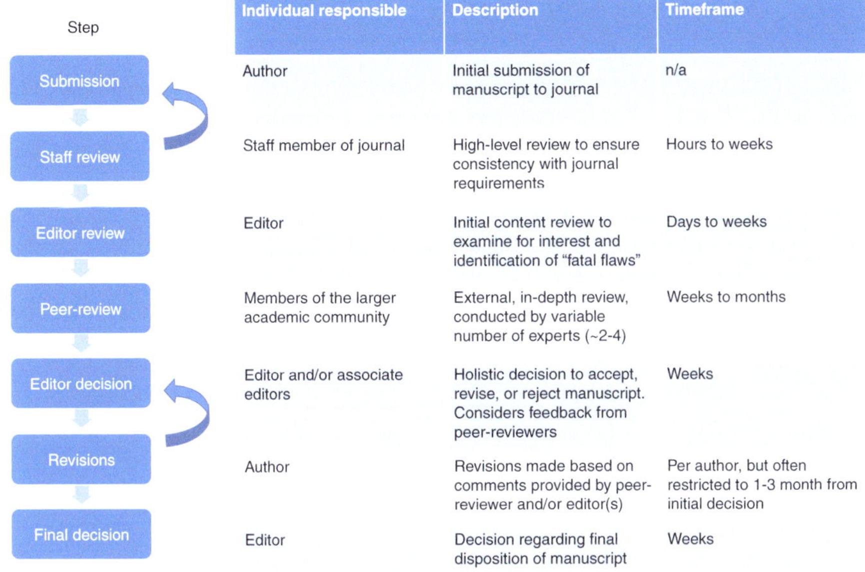

Fig. 13.2 The typical stages of peer review at a journal

13.2.1 Step 1: The Submission

Before submitting a manuscript, make sure that you understand the requirements of the journal, the guidelines, and the process your manuscript will take along its peer-review path. This pre-submission check is particularly important to ensure the quality of the journal and the integrity of the peer-review process of the journal. Whether a journal is subscription based or open access, the peer-review process should be equally as stringent. However, some journals are known as predatory or pseudo-journals that take advantage of authors and have suboptimal peer-review practices.

Beware of submitting to a journal that employs any of the following red flag signs of predatory practices:

- Soliciting the manuscript by spam email
- Unusually short submission-to-publication time (e.g., weeks)
- The website does not specify the peer-review process
- Charging a fee* for submission or the peer review

*Note: fees for publication, known as article processing charges (APCs), are not considered predatory. APCs should be transparent and known to the author up front. However, authors should not be charged for peer review or submission of a manuscript.

13.2.2 Step 2: The Staff Review

The peer-review process typically begins immediately after the submission of the manuscript. Within a few hours to several days, a high-level review of the manuscript is conducted by the journal, typically a staff member. In this phase of the review, the staff member considers the format of the manuscript and looks for inconsistencies between the journal requirements and the submission. Examples of this can include incorrect labeling of sections or unacceptable file formats. Usually, if there are issues at this stage, the author will have the opportunity to make appropriate revisions and resubmit. It is also possible for a manuscript to be rejected outright at this stage. Therefore, authors need to check formatting guidelines before they submit.

13.2.3 Step 3: The Editor's First Pass

Following the initial screening process, a manuscript is then considered by the editor or, in some cases, an associate editor. The purpose of this first-level review is to identify a subset of manuscripts that warrant peer review. In this stage, the editor considers the overall fitness of the manuscript for the journal in question. Fitness might include:

- Congruence with the journal's mission
- The importance of the topic for the target audience
- The timeliness of the subject matter
- The quality of how the work was carried out

For a few journals, this step is a formality, because nearly all manuscripts are sent for peer review. More commonly, editors receive more submissions than they can send for peer review, so they reject a significant portion of manuscripts at this stage.

Rejection before formal peer review is commonly described as the *desk reject*, suggesting that the manuscript was rejected from further consideration before it even left the desk of the editor. While a rejection at this early stage can feel defeating or may lead to challenges with a junior writer's confidence, there are at least two bright spots. First, the "desk reject" is generally relatively speedy. In our experience (and yes, we have all experienced desk rejects), the turnaround time ranges from a few hours to a few weeks. Though it may be vexing to have hard work readily dismissed, the swiftness allows writers the opportunity to move on to the next journal equally apace. Second, editors might provide feedback at this stage. While in some cases the comments are generic, i.e., "We receive many submissions and cannot accommodate them all," in other cases, there are concrete, actionable comments that the author can consider incorporating before submitting the manuscript to a different journal.

If a manuscript survives the desk reject stage, it then moves to the peer-review stage. Some journals actively notify authors at this point of the review cycle, while other journals only provide updates on a web space that authors need to actively check or give no notification at all. If an author is notified that their manuscript has made it past the editor's desk and onto peer review, they can share the good news with co-authors and mentors.

13.2.4 Step 4: The Peer-Review Stage

For manuscripts that survive the desk reject, the next step is peer review. In some disciplines, the peer reviewer is called a *referee* but in many medical journals, they are simply called peer reviewers. The number of reviewers varies widely across journals. Most journals aim for two to four. Frequently, 1–2 of the reviewers are content experts, while an additional reviewer may be asked to provide input on methodology or analysis.

Peer reviewers are identified from three primary sources:

- The journal editorial board members
- Journal peer-review pool of experts in content/subject matter
- Individuals identified by the author

Editorial board members may be asked to review manuscripts based on their area of expertise and/or as a core requirement of their responsibilities as members of the board. External reviewers are typically volunteers who may be identified by the journal such as authors of accepted manuscripts or known content experts who volunteer to peer review through a self-nomination process.

There is often an option for authors to nominate peer reviewers. If the journal provides the option to nominate reviewers for your manuscript, we suggest that you enter names if you have any in mind. As the expert, you know the content best so might be acquainted with individuals who are well versed on the topic. Such reviewers are more likely to appreciate the importance of the work and will be able to provide both meaningful and constructive feedback. Additionally, peer reviewers are generally in short supply, so suggesting reviewers might help the journal find a match for your manuscript more quickly and thereby decrease the time between your submission and initial decision.

For the reasons above, we encourage authors to nominate potential peer reviewers but with a few caveats. First, you should only nominate individuals who will have no conflict reviewing your work. A peer review should never come from within your institution, and a reviewer should never feel compelled to complete a biased review. Second, you should choose peer reviewers wisely. If your manuscript directly contradicts the work of another researcher, you may want to consider whether that person is an appropriate selection even if they are an expert in the field. While anyone feeling conflicted ought to recuse themselves, you want to avoid placing a colleague in a precarious situation. Third, if you do not have anyone to suggest, do not anguish. Some journals are open about the fact that they do not use the reviewers who are suggested by the authors, so do not go out of your way just to find reviewers' names to write down.

13.2.4.1 What Is in a Peer Review

Most, if not all, educational journals provide detailed guidelines for peer reviewers. These often include specific instructions on elements to address in the review, requirements for formulating a summary recommendation, and specific anchors to help guide the assessment of the manuscript. There are nuances to the format of a given review that may be based on the journal itself, or often, the type of manuscript that is being reviewed.

While the variation in requirements is quite diverse, there are five critical questions each reviewer is generally asked to address:

1. Is the manuscript important?
2. Was the approach (method) appropriate?
3. Was the authors' interpretation of the results appropriate?
4. What is the impact?
5. Is there alignment among the sections?

Importance. No educator would spend time writing about a subject if they did not feel it was important, so let us clarify what we mean by importance. Importance is about value. It is how much/how well the manuscript contributes to the existing body of literature.

- Is the manuscript timely?
- Does it fill a gap in the existing literature?
- How relevant is the gap for educational or clinical practice?

Approach. This consideration deals specifically with the methods selected and the alignment with the research question. For example, the description of a phenomenon commonly requires a qualitative methodology; meanwhile, an examination of performance between two groups necessitates an experimental or quasi-experimental design. In this consideration, the reviewer considers both the high-level alignment (e.g., question aligned with design) and the details (e.g., statistical analysis aligned with the sample).

Interpretation. The introduction and discussion sections provide an opportunity to share both perspective and interpretation. Without these sections, there is no purpose to the study, and there is no meaning in the results. However, one must be cautious, particularly in the discussion section. The discussion should relate to the purpose and should not overstate what was found in the study. In considering the interpretation, a peer reviewer considers whether the conclusions the authors offer are based on the study at hand. Failure to provide a reasonable interpretation, which includes reflection on key limitations, is critical.

Impact. All manuscripts should answer the "who cares" question. The authors found X …but does it matter? Related to the concept of importance, impact considers the educational impact of the manuscript. It is not necessary for every paper to fundamentally change the landscape of clinical or educational practice, but there must be some larger value to the contribution than simply an interesting finding.

Alignment. Finally, the peer reviewer considers alignment. As alluded to above in the discussion around approach, questions must align with methods, methods align with results, and the whole manuscript provides a well-thought-out narrative. Cohesion between sections, or the lack thereof, is a common reason for manuscript acceptance or rejection.

13.2.5 Step 5: The Editor's Decision

Once peer reviews are completed, they are compiled and shared with the editor to make an initial decision. It is critical to recognize that the editor's decision is exactly that; it is up to the editor to make the decision.

Peer reviews are invaluable to help guide the decision, but the editor is generally not required to follow the recommendations of the peer-reviewer. This point is crucial in helping junior writers reconcile why a peer reviewer's comments may be glowing, yet the final decision may still be unfavorable. When the editor decides, various factors can weigh in including reviewers' expertise, quality of the reviews, knowledge of the literature, journal interest in the particular subject, novelty of the work, and other factors.

Most journals provide a variety of decision options that include outright rejection, major revisions, minor revisions, and acceptance. However, for all practical purposes, there are essentially two decisions at this point: *reject* or *revise*.

Rejection: Rejections are unfortunately common in medical education research. However, they are also not the end of the world nor do they need to be the end of the line for a manuscript. If your manuscript has made it past the point of peer review to a final decision of rejection, you will be provided with peer-review comments that hold a wealth of useful feedback. There are often also comments from the editor. Comments and suggestions from reviewers and the editor should be considered a highly valuable resource that can be used to improve the manuscript before it is submitted to a different journal.

Revision: An invitation to revise a manuscript is a positive response even though these letters often come with the caveat that publication is not guaranteed. In our experience, an outright acceptance on the first pass is extremely rare. Therefore, the most realistic positive outcome of an initial manuscript submission is the invitation to revise the manuscript for resubmission.

13.2.6 *Step 6: The Revision*

The difference between major and minor revisions is to a degree semantic. Historically, *major revisions* meant that there was a significant need to rework sections, introduce new concepts, and/or reconsider analysis. A *minor revision* meant that there were less significant changes needed to the substance of the manuscript. More recently, however, we have found that almost all initial revisions are characterized with the term "major revision" and the term "minor revision" is used for extremely small typographical errors or formatting issues.

An author should be less concerned about whether the revision was labeled as *minor* or *major* and instead focus attention on implementing the suggested changes so that the resubmission can have the best chance of gaining acceptance. A request for revisions typically comes with unedited comments from peer reviewers, comments from the editor(s), and specific instructions regarding the format for submitting revisions including a timeline.

The author needs to consider all instructions and guidance provided by the journal at this point in the process. Each comment from peer reviewers and editors must be considered thoughtfully and must be discussed when submitting revisions. It is not necessary to make every change a reviewer suggests, but it is necessary to respond to each suggestion and provide justification (with evidence) if a change is not made. Additionally, the format for submitting revisions must be followed; some journals require a tabular format for submitting revisions while others expect a narrative summary.

Scholarship is difficult, and receiving criticism on your hard work is not easy. When critical peer-review feedback first arrives, it is not uncommon to feel some amount of personal affront. A reviewer's comments can initially feel biting and vexing, even if they are meant to be helpful and respectful. When this happens, take time to let the reality of the situation settle—an offer to revise is a cause for celebration and peer reviewers are offering advice to strengthen the manuscript—and then read the reviewer comments one at a time. Try to remember that reviewers are equivalent to your intended audience. If the peer reviewer did not understand a message or concept being conveyed in the manuscript, then the readership of the journal also will not understand the message or concept as it was written. A peer reviewer that has volunteered time to read your work and offered their suggestions for improvements has done you a service. For these collegial offerings, we need to maintain a grateful attitude. Anger or frustration with the peer reviewer is unhelpful at best. Passive-aggressive remarks to the editor or in the response have no place. When writing the response letter, it might be necessary to make multiple passes through before submitting it to ensure that any discourteous tone is removed. Having a friendly colleague read through the responses can also help ensure that remarks are appropriately respectful.

Once revisions have been submitted, the editor has the option of circulating the manuscript for additional review or deciding the manuscript's disposition on their own. In our experience, we have seen both used. The former, sending for another cycle of peer review, is typically used when there are issues that are contentious such as those that might affect broader policy, theoretical discussions, or issues that require additional analysis, and the editor feels that there is a benefit from hearing additional voices to help with the decision. The editor might instead decide the manuscript's disposition on their own if the initial reviewer comments were more clarification based and well addressed by the author in the response letter.

As shown in Fig. 13.3, the process for revisions and re-review may continue for several rounds. In the best-case scenario, an initial decision of "major revision" is

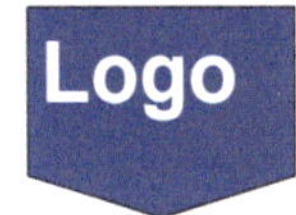

Date

Journal Name

Dear Editorial Staff,

We are pleased to resubmit our manuscript entitled "Fabulous Study of High Importance: On Topic Related to Education Scholarship" for consideration as an article for publication in the journal.

In response to the editorial office reviewer comments, we have amended the manuscript. Please see below for specific responses to the reviewer comments.

> *Reviewer #1: In Line 10 regarding...//... I feel this is not appropriate or accurate.*
>
>> **Our Response:** We recognize that this is a contentious issue and raises conflicts between...//.... To soften this, we have removed the word () and changed to sentence to read: "...//..."
>>
>> We hope you find this wording acceptable.
>
> *Reviewer #1: On p. 11, line 46, remove the words ....*
>
>> **Our Response:** We appreciate these comments by Reviewer #1. We have removed the wording from the manuscript.
>
> *Reviewer #2: I applaud the authors ...//....*
>
>> **Our Response:** Thank you for your comments.
>
> *Reviewer #2: This is an issue that has significant impacts...//... the last two sentences in the conclusion of this paper would make a good starting point for a rewrite.*
>
>> **Our Response:** We appreciate the reviewer pointing out...//... In the introduction, we added...//... Within the section on (), we have further emphasized the role of...//... We agree that these are interesting areas for exploration and potential research, but further elaboration on these issues would be beyond the scope of this paper and be detrimental to maintaining an appropriate manuscript length. To further address the concern raised of (), we have reworked the information regarding (). In the section applying (), we have added more specific suggestions for...//... To further address the issues raised regarding rewriting the paper, we have significantly expanded and reworked our conclusions with () that can be created to better address these important issues.
>
> *Reviewer #2: On page 3, line 33 - I've never seen...//...; recommend revising this to read...//.... I would also make ...//... read as ...//....*
>
>> **Our Response:** We appreciate the discerning comments of Review #2. We have incorporated these changes.
>
> *Reviewer #2: I have a problem with the statement on page 10, line 43. As written, it implies...//....*
>
>> **Our Response (as above):** We recognize that this is a contentious issue and raises conflicts between (). To soften this, we have removed the word () and changed to sentence to read: ...//... We hope you find this wording acceptable.

We are grateful for these very helpful comments by the reviewing staff of the Journal. The insightful comments were instrumental in guiding the authors to producing a clearer and more poignant manuscript. We hope you will be pleased and satisfied with the changes we have made since receiving the comments. We respectfully resubmit our manuscript to you for consideration.

This manuscript has not been previously published and is not under consideration in the same or substantially similar form in any other peer-reviewed media.

All authors listed have contributed sufficiently to the project to be included as authors, and all those who are qualified to be authors are listed in the author byline. To the best of our knowledge, no conflict of interest, financial or other, exists.

Sincerely,

You R. Scholar

Fig. 13.3 Sample revision response letter

downgraded to a "minor revision" or to an acceptance. However, the journal could also require additional major revisions or reject the manuscript. We have found additional revisions common when issues could impact policy and small nuances in wording could lead to a large impact on implementation. Rejection is most common when authors inadequately address or ignore the comments of a reviewer, and this consequence highlights the importance of carefully considering and addressing each and every comment made by a reviewer during the revision process.

13.2.7 Final Decision

At some point in the process, the editor will issue a final decision—accept or reject. And in virtually all cases, the final decision is final. There may be occasions in which an author can appeal a decision, but this is extremely rare. If the decision is positive, share the good news with your colleagues and celebrate. The journal will contact you with the next steps. If the decision is "reject," carefully consider any comments from the journal editor or peer reviewers, so you can incorporate the feedback as you move forward.

13.3 Giving Back to the Peer-Review Process

Every health scholar ought to consider being active in the peer-review process for academic journals. Peer reviewers provide a valuable contribution to the scientific community, and this important task needs a representation of scholars from a diversity of backgrounds including diversity of gender, race, academic rank, and geographic location to ensure that the outcomes are just and equitable. By serving as peer reviewers, scholars serve their community by performing quality checks on manuscripts to catch any issues with methods, analysis, or conclusions before the research is published.

Service is a key component of the peer-review system, but there are also benefits to the individual scholar. While helping others, writing creativity is stimulated and this can help the health scholar start or continue their own writing efforts. Peer-review work also helps to demystify the academic publishing process. Many journals provide peer reviewers with detailed comments offered by all reviewers and the final decision rendered by the journal. By both critiquing the work of others and reflecting on the final decision, authors can be better informed about the type of work that is accepted or rejected. This information can be instrumental in informing one's own scholarly writing.

With the transformations in publication and increase in the number of peer-reviewed journals, there are ample opportunities to volunteer as a reviewer. Editors are faced with an increased need for reviewers, so they value scholars willing to volunteer their time and ability. Reviewing is considered an important contribution to a clinician-educator curriculum vitae (CV) since service is commonly valued for promotion and tenure decisions. In addition to listing the service on your CV, many journals now track peer reviewers and recognize reviewers annually in their publications or a special report. Some provide awards to those who deliver consistently strong (helpful) reviews.

In a 2016 survey of peer reviewers asking why they performed reviews, their answers fell into the following categories [5]:

Social factors:

- To play a part as a member of the community (93%)
- To help others improve their papers (83%)
- To reciprocate for others reviewing work (75%)
- Enjoyment of seeing work ahead of publication (72%)

Self-interested factors:

- Enhancement of career (42%)
- Possibility of editorial board (24%)
- Increase the chance of future acceptance (16%)

13.3.1 Process for Becoming a Peer Reviewer

There are two main ways to become a peer reviewer, by self-nomination or by invitation. First, you can self nominate to be a peer reviewer. The website of most major journals includes a section for prospective peer reviewers to indicate interest in serving. This often includes an opportunity to indicate content expertise, thus enabling editors to identify the most applicable manuscripts for assignment to individuals. In the second option, a request to peer review comes to you directly from a journal. This might occur if an author identifies you as a content expert at the time they submit a manuscript, and the journal decides to pursue you as the peer reviewer.

Peer reviewers should be content experts, and junior scholars may wonder if they have the experience or expertise to serve in this role. One way to mitigate this challenge is to participate in a mentored peer review. Increasingly, journals permit and even encourage senior peer reviewers to include a junior member or a team of junior members in their reviews of a manuscript. If journals do not explicitly encourage or invite these types of team reviews, we have found that most journals are agreeable if a request is sent in writing to the journal staff.

Training for peer review is also offered through academic societies, research academies, and major publishers. Many of these resources are offered for free and can be found through internet search engines using terms such as "peer review training courses." Some allow access without a log-in, while others use log-ins and allow linking to institutional credentialing systems. There are also articles on how to peer review. These are available with general guidelines such as Azer's 2012 article [6] or guidelines that are specifically geared to specialty journals. Using search terms "Peer Review" and "how-to" plus your specialty journal name(s) can help you find an article specific to your academic field or journal of interest.

It usually takes only a few peer reviews to start feeling comfortable with the process of peer reviewing. The learning curve is assisted by doing a review and then receiving the editor's comments, final decision, and copy of other peer reviews performed on the same manuscript. This affords the peer reviewer the opportunity to retrospectively compare their comments to other reviewers' comments.

13.3.2 Peer-Review Caution

It can be professionally satisfying to complete a peer review for a journal and thereby offer service to the community. However, there are some notes of caution. Once a journal finds a peer reviewer who is reliable and responsive, it is common for the journal to continue to send review invitations. Often, as soon as one review is complete, the next invitation arrives. While flattering, it can feel as if a flood gate of invitations to review manuscripts and a time sink of uncompensated work have suddenly taken hold of your calendar. At first, it is good to get involved in peer reviewing others, learning the system, and getting practice, but there needs to be a balance between your service to a journal and your time spent writing for publication. For every one manuscript that you submit to a journal, the journal will need help reviewing several manuscripts in return, and the number varies based on the journal. However, if you find that you are peer reviewing frequently but making no manuscript submissions, it might be time to reconsider priorities and set aside more writing time for your own endeavors.

It is imperative that you feel comfortable turning down peer reviews:

- When you do not have the time
- When there is a conflict of interest
- If the topic is unfamiliar or not in your area of expertise

Caution regarding confidentiality vs. transparency: Journals differ on how much information reviewers are given regarding authors and whether authors are given information regarding who has reviewed their work. In an effort to reduce bias, some journals mask the names of the authors and the reviewers. However, to improve transparency, some journals identify both authors and reviewers; they might even publish the review along with the paper when it is published, e.g., "open review." Open reviews can help temper reviewer comments, making them kinder and less harsh; however, they also can put a reviewer at risk if there is a power differential between the reviewer and author. Open reviews have the advantage of holding the reviewer accountable for the scientific integrity of the paper; however, they can also hold the reviewer liable for the social aspects of an article once it is published.

13.4 Conclusion

The peer-review process is critical to the production of educational scholarship. Although peer review is an imperfect process, it has helped improve the quality of published papers for the past 300 years. Even when manuscripts are rejected after going through the peer-review process, the comments from reviewers often provide useful feedback. Participating in the peer-review process as a reviewer is also advantageous to demystify the academic publishing process, stimulate one's own writing, and be an active member of the scientific community. By better understanding the steps involved in peer review, we hope that you are better able to construct educational manuscripts for publication.

13.5 Questions

Activities

1. Identify a journal in which you have published or aim to publish your work. Investigate whether they accept self-nominations for peer review. If so, sign up!
2. Trade manuscripts with a colleague. Complete a mock peer review using the included peer review template.

Peer review template:

Component	Prompt	Impression		Comments
		Yes	No	
Title				
	Is the title clear, informative, and does it represent the content?	☐	☐	
Question, Annotated bibliography, Logistics, mentor Reflection				
	Is the problem clearly and logically stated in the question?	☐	☐	
	Does the annotated bibliography identify a gap and formulate the basis for study?	☐	☐	
	Does the list of logistics show a comprehensive consideration of resources?	☐	☐	
	Does the mentor narrative reflect insights into potential barriers to implementation of the educational project?	☐	☐	
Learning Outcomes, Educational Methods, and Evaluation Design				
	Is the conceptual framework explicit and justified?	☐	☐	
	Are the learning outcomes attainable, and do they flow from the scholarship question?			
	Is there congruency between the scholarship question, educational methods, evaluation design, and outcomes?	☐	☐	
	Is the evaluation design appropriate for the project outcomes?	☐	☐	

Component	Prompt	Impression		Comments
		Yes	No	
	Is the approach/are the aspired outcomes likely to be generalizable/of more than local relevance?	☐	☐	
IRB Considerations				
	Are all potential risks and benefits to project participants identified and balanced?	☐	☐	
	Are appropriate measures suggested to protect vulnerable human subjects' rights?	☐	☐	
Abstract				
	Are the authors appropriately listed?	☐	☐	
	Is the abstract length and organizational subdivision into purpose and methods sections well chosen?	☐	☐	
	Does the *Methods* section state the design or protocol right away and give the who, where, when, and how?	☐	☐	
Presentation				
	Is the text well written and easy to follow?	☐	☐	
	Is the paper well organized?	☐	☐	
Summary Comments				

References

1. Spier R. The history of the peer-review process. Trends Biotechnol. 2002;20(8):357–8.
2. Richlin L. Scholarly teaching and the scholarship of teaching. New directions for teaching and learning. 2001. pp. 57–68.
3. Glassick CE. Boyer's expanded definition of scholarship, the standards for assessing scholarship, and the elusiveness of the scholarship of teaching. Acad Med. 2000;75:877–80.
4. During SJ, Carline JD, editors. Review criteria for research manuscripts. 2nd ed. Washington: Association of American Medical Colleges; 2015.
5. Publishing Research Consortium. Publishing research consortium peer review survey 2015. London: Mark Ware Consulting; 2016.
6. Azer SA, Ramani S, Peterson R. Becoming a peer reviewer to medical education journals. Medical Teacher. 2012;34(9):698–704.

Part V
Behind the Scenes

Chapter 14
Project Planning and Logistics

Bonnie L. Robeson and April S. Fitzgerald

14.1 Introduction

Education scholarship is involved. Projects have multiple simultaneously operating components and steps to take a concept or idea from its stated objective to a published article or presentation. Navigating efficiently through the phases from research implementation to dissemination requires an organized logistical plan. While taking time at the start of a project to undertake detailed planning may at first seem like an unnecessary hindrance, forging ahead without thinking through the process is a certain way to cause backtracking and delays.

Project planning can start as an early activity once the topic idea is written out in a concise statement. Even at this early point, it is a good idea to think about the entire process including the endpoint   the stakeholders/readers whom the results of the scholarship are meant to reach and impact. Keep in mind that it is human nature to underestimate the amount of time a project, research, or scholarly research publication will take.

Previous chapters introduced basic concepts of educational scholarship and its importance in disseminating innovative concepts to colleagues. The first step is to form a research hypothesis, which leads to a research objective. Honing a concise overarching objective statement is essential. The next steps include a literature review and formulating the project. Identifying the audience for the project outcome

B. L. Robeson (✉)
The Johns Hopkins Carey Business School, Baltimore, MD, USA
e-mail: brobeson@jhu.edu

A. S. Fitzgerald
Division of General Internal Medicine, Department of Medicine, Johns Hopkins University School of Medicine, Baltimore, MD, USA
e-mail: afitzg10@jhmi.edu

205

A. S. Fitzgerald, G. Bosch (eds.), *Education Scholarship in Healthcare*, https://doi.org/10.1007/978-3-031-38534-6_14

and understanding the stakeholders will assist in the journal and/or conference selection.

This chapter discusses organization as the key to a smooth process of implementing an education project. Being organized emphasizes thinking ahead. It is also important to understand that not every activity will go as planned.

Several project tools can be used in the planning phase:

- Cause and effect—the logic model
- Project overview—PERT/Gantt charts
- Budget and expenses—budget/expense templates
- Resources—resource planning template

14.2 Project Cause and Effect: The Logic Model

A *logic model* graphicly depicts cause and effects in the chain of events that lead from project start to project completion. Using a model can help aid in understanding the relationship of activities as they occur in sequence. They can serve to confirm the thought process and the logic of a project hypothesis, or they can identify flaws or gaps in the logic allowing these deficiencies to be corrected. A logic model can also help identify assumptions. By tying the original research idea to the final report for publication, there is less room for projects to venture off target.

Many templates for logic models are available for free online or one can be constructed by hand. A sample template is presented in Table 14.1, and an example model is shown in Fig. 14.1. A well-developed logic model can pay off for the health scholar through the improved alignment of research objectives with data evaluation and the intended impact [1]. Understanding each column in the logic model—Purpose, Objective/Hypothesis, Stakeholders/Audience, Resources, Short-term Outcomes, Medium- to Long-term Outcomes, and Impact—is essential for the project. Logic models can also be used for structuring the final article, and a few sentences from each category can be used to compose the manuscript abstract.

Table 14.1 Logic model template

Objective/Hypothesis	Activities	OUTCOMES		
		Short-term	Medium/Long term	Impact

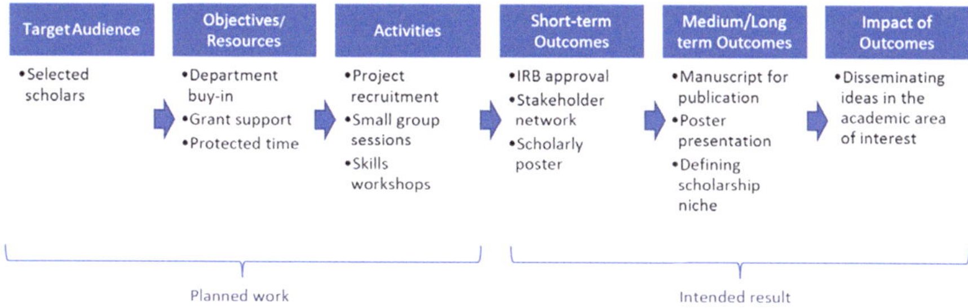

Fig. 14.1 Example logic model

Fig. 14.2 PERT chart vs. Gantt chart

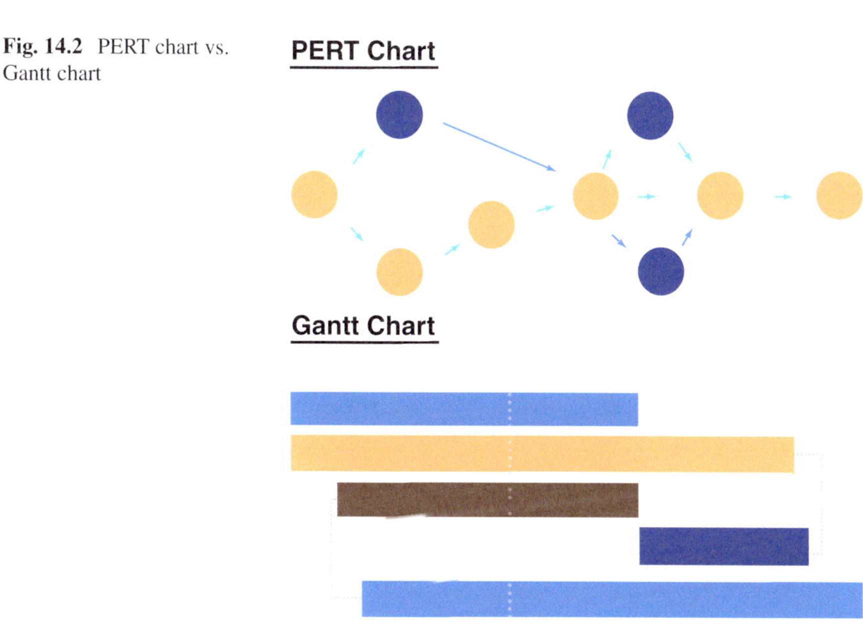

14.3   Project Overview: Gantt/PERT Charts

Gantt charts, named for Henry Gantt who popularized their use in the early twentieth century, track tasks using bar graphs to track percent completion. *PERT (Program Evaluation and Review Technique) charts*, in contrast, are flow diagrams and offer a simplified visual guide for tracking a project plan (Fig. 14.2).

PERT originated in the late 1950s by Navy government contractors [2]. The purpose of the technique was to track and keep large projects on time. Since government contractors often have subcontractors and sub-subcontractors, it is important for large projects with tens of thousands of tasks being conducted by numerous contractors to come together to meet time constraints. PERT is now considered one of the most useful and used management science tools.

Education scholarship is well suited to use these charts due to the nature of a *project*. Each project is a one-of-a-kind, unique undertaking. Each educational research project will have its own uniqueness that must be recognized—even though it may have commonalities with other research publication projects conducted in the past. Therefore, it is important to take past experience and combine that information with newer unknown factors.

The PERT method has the following characteristics:

- Probabilistic (based on chance variation)
- Visual
- Shows critical path
- Adjustable

After careful selection of a medical education scholarship topic, the health scholar will want to start considering the steps that are necessary to carry out the intended project.

The following aspects of a project can be visualized by a PERT chart, so should be considered in the project planning phase:

- Expected time for completion of the overall project
- Activities that can be conducted simultaneously
- Activities whose start is dependent on another activity's completion
- Activities with slack time (adjustable start or completion time)
- Activities that must be started and completed on time or else risk project delay
- An activity's optimistic timeline, most likely timeline, and pessimistic timeline

Health scholars can either use their own experience, ask for mentor/colleague input, or seek historical data to help with estimates when attempting to gauge the timelines for their project and the timelines for activities within the project. Doing this type of projection is essential for projects working with a firm deadline.

14.3.1 Creating a PERT Chart

PERT charts are composed of nodes and arches between nodes that create a network. One method is to put the activities on the arches, but more often, the activities are on the nodes.

The basic steps in conducting an analysis to create a PERT chart are the following:

Step 1: List your project activities from the initial project start to the conclusion. In the case of an educational scholarship project, the conclusion will be some form of dissemination such as the publication of an article.

Step 2: For each activity in step 1, indicate if there are any immediate predecessor activities, e.g., what task must be completed before that activity can start. This step will define dependencies and later allow visualization by connecting and numbering/lettering activities.

Step 3: Determine how long each activity is expected to take. Each activity's time is estimated in three different ways—optimistic (T_o), most likely (T_m), and pessimistic (T_p).

- *Optimistic time* is the time required when everything for the activity proceeds as planned.
- *Most likely time* is the average time for that activity.
- *Pessimistic time* estimates time accounting for almost everything being delayed

    All activities must be in the same time unit, such as hours, days, or weeks. It is best to use the smallest unit of time to avoid rounding errors. A note of caution regarding querying others for help in time estimation: there is skill and art required for stating the question. The question needs to be stated in a way that will obtain honest information rather than being told what the person thinks you *want* to hear.

    Next, determine the *expected time* for each activity:

$$\text{Activity expected time} = \left(T_o + \left(4 \times T_m \right) + T_p \right) \div 6.$$

The optimistic time (T_o) and pessimistic time (T_p) are given a weight of one (1), while the most likely time (T_m) is given a weight of four (4). The sum of these estimated time components is then divided by six (6) to give a weighted average, which is a beta distribution.

Step 4: Draw the network.

- List the first activity as a node, and connect it to the next node (activity) using an arrow.
- Continue placing nodes for subsequent activities with arrows to indicate dependencies and connections.
- The chart (and arrows) should flow from left to right; try to avoid vertical arrows. The final node of the PERT chart is the project conclusion.
- Calculate *earliest start* (ES) and *earliest finish* (EF) by going left to right in a forward pass.
- *earliest start* = the earliest date when a task can start (dependent task must be completed)
- *earliest finish* = earliest start + activity duration
- Calculate the *latest start* (LS) and *latest finish* (LF) by going right to left in a backward pass.
- *latest start* = last-day activity can start without delaying the project
- *latest finish* = last-day activity can finish without delaying the project
- Calculate *activity* slack time
- *slack time* = (*latest finish* − *earliest finish*) or (*latest start* − *earliest start*)
- Trace the project critical path: LF = EF. The critical path is the one where slack is zero for activities.

When making a PERT chart, it is not unusual to go through multiple iterations.

14.3.2 *Example PERT Chart for a Scholarly Project*

Let us look at a PERT example for a generic scholarly project.

First, a small example will be used to explain in detail each sequential step. Then, a more realistic multistep example using software to assist with the calculations will be presented.

14.3.2.1 Small Project Example: Creating a PERT Chart

Step 1: List all activities in the project. For this example, we will use a small project with only nine steps labeled A through I; see Table 14.2, columns I and II.

Step 2: For each activity in step 1, determine the relationship between the activities. Predecessor activities must be completed before another activity can take place. Indicate if there are any immediate predecessors; see Table 14.2, column VIII.

Table 14.2 Small project tasks

I	II	III	IV	V	VI	VII	VIII
Activity	Activity task	Optimistic time (T_o)	Most likely time (T_m)	Pessimistic time (T_p)	Calculation of expected time $\left(\dfrac{To+(4\times Tm)+Tp}{6} \right)$	Expected time	Predecessor activities
A	Select topic	1	2	3	$\left(\dfrac{1+(4\times 2)+3}{6} \right)$	2	None
B	Conduct literature search	1	3	17	$\left(\dfrac{1+(4\times 3)+6}{6} \right)$	5	A
C	Hire researchers	3	8	13	$\left(\dfrac{3+(4\times 8)+13}{6} \right)$	8	A
D	Develop research procedure	2	2	2	$\left(\dfrac{2+(4\times 2)+2}{6} \right)$	2	B
E	Conduct research	4	10	22	$\left(\dfrac{4+(4\times 10)+22}{6} \right)$	11	C, D
F	Evaluate data	1	1	1	$\left(\dfrac{1+(4\times 1)+1}{6} \right)$	1	E
G	Evaluate journals for submission	2	5	32	$\left(\dfrac{2+(4\times 5)+32}{6} \right)$	9	F
H	Write article	1	3	5	$\left(\dfrac{1+(4\times 3)+5}{6} \right)$	3	F
I	Publish article	4	4	4	$\left(\dfrac{4+(4\times 4)+4}{6} \right)$	4	H

Step 3: Determine how long each activity is expected to take—optimistic (T_o), most likely (T_m), and pessimistic (T_p). Determine these three times for each activity either from past data or by judgment; see Table 14.2, columns III, IV, and V. Optimistic time (T_o) is the time if everything goes at maximum efficiency. Most likely time (T_m) is how long an activity takes to perform the majority of the time. Pessimistic time (T_p) is the worst-case scenario when everything goes wrong. All times must be in the same unit. Therefore, one activity cannot be in days and another in weeks. It is best to convert all times to the lowest value. This will avoid rounding errors. For this example, the time period used will be defined as 1 week.

Next, determine the *expected time* for each activity: $\left(\dfrac{To+(4\times Tm)+Tp}{6}\right)$. See Table 14.2, column VI.

Example using activity E:

Calculate the activity expected time for activity "E" of "Select Data" using the given optimistic, most likely, and pessimistic times from the table.

Remember that the formula is a weighted average with "most likely time" given a weight of 4, the other times given a weight of 1, and the denominator being always six (the weights added together, $(1 + 4 + 1 = 6)$).

Expected

$$\text{time} = \left(\frac{(1)(\text{optimistic time})+(4)(\text{most likely time})+(1)(\text{pessimistic time})}{1+4+1}\right)$$

Expected time of activity

$$E = \left(\frac{(1)(4)+(4)(10)+(1)(22)}{6}\right) = \left(\frac{(4)+(40)+22)}{6}\right) = \left(\frac{(66)}{6}\right)$$

Expected time activity $E = 11$

Step 4: Draw the network using the predecessor activities. Once drawn, no activity should be left without a connection to the final finish node. The network should have a direction of left to right and should avoid using perpendicular lines.

Below is a node that represents a single activity. The upper-left cell is the *activity name*. The top-right cell is for the calculated expected time of the activity (Fig. 14.3).

Enter calculated expected times in the upper right cell. Look at the diagram, and make a forward pass moving from left to right to calculate the earliest start (ES) and earliest finish (EF). The earliest time starts at zero (ES = 0) for activity A, and then you add the expected time to ES to yield the EF (earliest finish) time for the activity.

Figure 14.4 shows an example of how to start the left-to-right pass along the PERT diagram works. Only columns I, VII, and VIII of the previously created (Table 14.2) chart are needed for this left-to-right pass. When two activities feed into one node, it is the larger of the two numbers (longer time) which is used since the activity can only start when both predecessor activities have been completed. For example, nodes C and D feed into node E, so the later start time is used. Therefore, the earliest start time for node E is 10.

Fig. 14.3 Node construct

Activity Name	Expected Time
ES (Earliest Start)	**EF** (Earliest Finish)
LS (Late Start)	**LF** (Late Finish)
s (slack)	

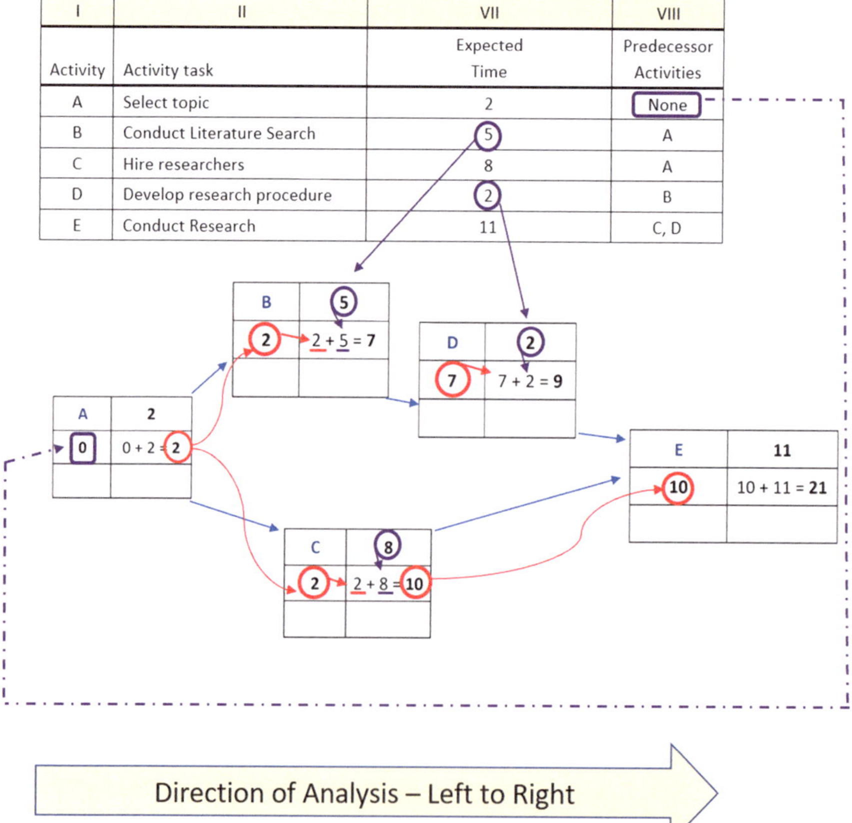

Fig. 14.4 Partial forward pass (left to right) on PERT diagram using PERT chart

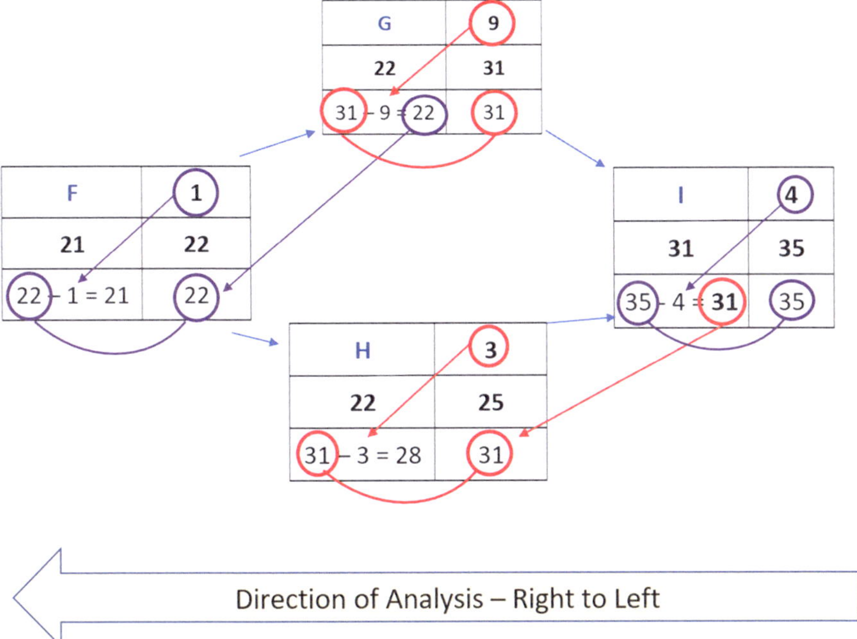

Fig. 14.5 Partial backward pass (right to left) on PERT diagram

Once the last node is calculated, the backward pass is made moving from right to left. Figure 14.5 shows an example of how to start the right-to-left pass along the PERT diagram. On the final node (I), set the latest finish (LF) equal to the earliest finish (EF).

Calculate latest start by subtracting the activity time from the latest finish time. For node I, 35–4 = 31. When two nodes feed into a single node (moving from right to left), then the smallest time is moved to the left into the latest finish (LF) position of the node. Continue working from right to left. For example: Looking at node F, the latest finish time is 22; you then subtract 1 (the expected activity time for activity F) to get the latest start time for F, which is 21.

The final step is to calculate slack. Slack is equal to latest finish (LF) minus the earliest finish (LF − EF) or the late start minus the early start (LS − ES). If calculations are different, then there is a math mistake. The critical path is determined by connecting the activities with zero slack. The critical path must connect from the start to the finish. This is always the longest path, and each of these activities must start and finish on time for the project to be completed by the earliest finish (EF) time. The critical path should be made evident by some means, either using double arrows as connectors, highlighting the nodes, or both as shown in Fig. 14.6.

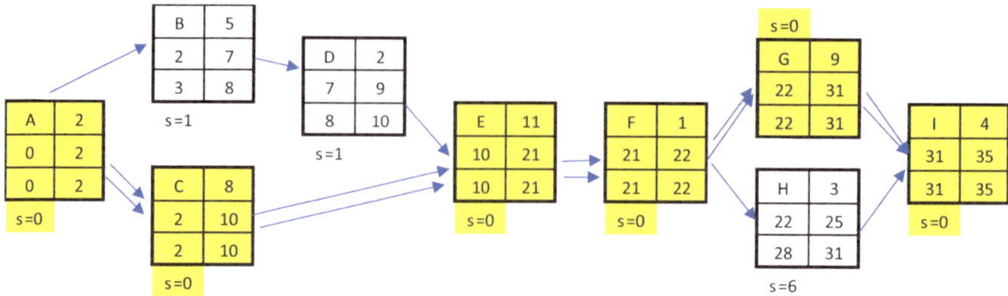

Fig. 14.6 Example small project PERT chart diagram

14.3.2.2 Small Project Example: Interpretation of the PERT Chart and Diagram

The expected time to complete the example small project is the number listed in the earliest finish (EF) position of the project's last node (I). This value for the small project is 35. Since the units of the project are all measured in weeks, the project expected time is 35 weeks. Three different projected times to completion were used—optimistic time, most likely time, and pessimistic time—so the result is a normal distribution meaning that 50% of the time the project will finish earlier than 35 weeks, and 50% of the time the project will take longer than 35 weeks.

The standard deviation for the project can be determined using the activities on the critical path. To determine the standard deviation, first calculate the variance for each activity on the critical path using the formula $(\delta^2) = \left(\text{Pessimistic time-Optimistic time}\right)^2 \Big/ 6^2$. Once the variance is calculated, the standard deviation is simply the square root of the variance.

As seen in Table 14.3, the variance for the critical pathway of the small project is 36.9. Let us round this down to 36. Standard deviation is the square root of variance. Therefore, the standard deviation for the project is the square root of 36 or approximately 6 (weeks).

Interpretation of the PERT standard deviation: Knowing the standard deviation, it can be said that two-thirds of the time (68% or one-standard deviation on either side of the mean), the project will be completed between 29 and 41 weeks, e.g., between (35 − 6 weeks) and (35 + 6 weeks); see Fig. 14.7.

14.3.2.3 Large Project Example: Creating a PERT Chart

Next, let us do a larger example that is more realistic of what you might do for an actual project. There will be 25 activities, and we will input these into a software program to compute the data. Using software makes it easier to adjust and recalculate the critical path as events occur that cause the *expected* times to change during the project or if a task runs late.

Table 14.3 Small project variance

Activity	Optimistic time (T_o)	Pessimistic time (T_p)	Variance $\left(Pessimistic\ time - Optimistic\ time\right)^2 / 6^2$
A	1	3	$\left(3-1\right)^2 / 6^2 = \left(2\right)^2 / 6^2 = 4/36$
C	3	13	$\left(13-3\right)^2 / 6^2 = \left(10\right)^2 / 6^2 = 100/36 =$
E	4	22	$\left(22-4\right)^2 / 6^2 = \left(18\right)^2 / 6^2 = 324/36 =$
F	1	1	$\left(1-1\right)^2 / 6^2 = -$
G	2	32	$\left(32-3\right)^2 / 6^2 = \left(30\right)^2 / 6^2 = 900/36 =$
I	4	4	$\left(4-4\right)^2 / 6^2 = -$
			$1328/36 = \mathbf{36.89}$

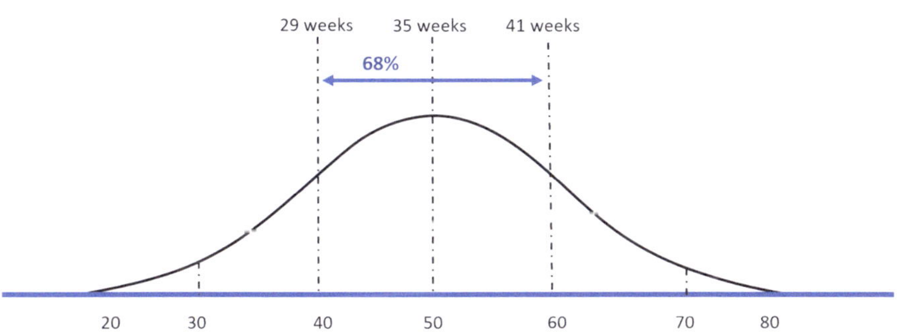

Fig. 14.7 Small project variance/standard deviation interpretation

Step 1: List project activities—see Table 14.4. Activities for this generic scholarly project are listed along column 2 and labeled in column 1 as items A through Y (25 activities). The concluding activity is the revision of the poster/article.

Step 2: See Table 14.5. For each activity A through Y of the scholarly project, the activity preceding it was determined and is listed in Table 14.5. Note that activities have more than one predecessor.

Step 3: See Table 14.5, columns 2–4. For this exercise, the chosen unit of time was days. For each activity, prior experience allowed columns 2, 3, and 4 to be filled in with the optimistic time (T_o), most likely time (T_m), and pessimistic time (T_p). For each activity, the activity expected time was then calculated with the formula $(To + (4 \times Tm) + Tp) \div 6$.

Step 4: Drawing the PERT chart. The diagram for the example scholarly project can now be drawn using the activities (items A–Y) as nodes. The nodes are

Table 14.4 Example project activities

Activity Label	Project activities
A	Formulate study objectives
B	Formulate study questions
C	Literature review
D	Experimental design
E	Develop methodology
F	Resources required
G	Budget
H	Funding request/grant applications
I	Develop curriculum/program
J	Review curriculum/program
K	Approval of curriculum/program
L	Advertise for assistants
M	Interview assistants
N	Hire or assign researchers
O	Acquire facilities/equipment
P	IRB application
Q	Recruit participants
R	Conduct program
S	Evaluate program
T	Select journal or conferences
U	Analyze data
V	Write article or poster
W	Submit article/poster
X	Revise article/poster
Y	Finish node

sometimes simplified to say activity 1 (or task), etc., but a more useful PERT chart has activity information contained in each node.

When drawing the PERT chart, activities do not occur in series as one item occurring after another. Instead, some items occur in parallel and are independent of other core activities but still feed into the final project endpoint. Note that now the immediate predecessors (dependencies) of Table 14.5 need to be considered when drawing the diagram, e.g., the study objectives (item A) must be determined before the experimental design (item D), and there must be resources (item F) before acquiring equipment (item O).

The expected start is the day after the prior (dependent) activity's end. For example, activity B starts one day after activity A finishes. The expected start for activity B is one day after activity A's expected time. The earliest start for activity B is one day after activity A's optimistic time (T_o), and activity B's latest start is one day after activity A's pessimistic time (T_p).

Table 14.5 PERT activities with predecessors and estimated times

Activity	Optimistic time	Most likely time	Pessimistic time	Predecessor 1	Predecessor 2	Predecessor 3	Predecessor 4	Predecessor 5	Predecessor 6	Predecessor 7
A	1	3	5							
B	2	4	6	A						
C	10	15	20	B						
D	5	12	19	A						
E	2	10	12	D						
F	4	8	12	E						
G	2	6	10	F						
H	10	30	56	G						
I	10	15	20	A	D					
J	15	20	25	I						
K	15	20	25	J						
L	4	8	12	G						
M	10	20	30	L						
N	10	15	32	M						
O	10	25	40	F	M					
P	14	20	44	K						
Q	12	30	66	P						
R	60	60	60	N	Q					
S	20	30	40	R						

(continued)

Table 14.5 (continued)

Activity	Optimistic time	Most likely time	Pessimistic time	Predecessor 1	Predecessor 2	Predecessor 3	Predecessor 4	Predecessor 5	Predecessor 6	Predecessor 7
T	5	10	15	S						
U	12	20	28	R						
V	5	15	25	U						
W	1	1	1	V						
X	4	8	12	W						
Y	0	0	0	C	H	O	S	T	W	X

Once the latest finish and earliest finish time are determined, the slack time can be calculated as (latest finish − earliest finish) (Figs. 14.8 and 14.9).

14.3.2.4   Large Project Example: Interpretation of the PERT Chart and Diagram

Now that the work of creating the PERT chart and PERT table has been completed, there is important information that can be gained from them. The overall diagram indicates the relationships among the activities.

Looking at the critical pathway, the expected time to complete the project from start to publication is the sum of the expected time it takes to complete the activities in the critical path. In this example, it is 230 weeks. This can be accomplished by adding up the times' columns where slack is zero. This time is at the second line of the table along with the standard deviation for the project. The red line indicates the critical path on the diagram. The values for the earliest start (ES), earliest finish

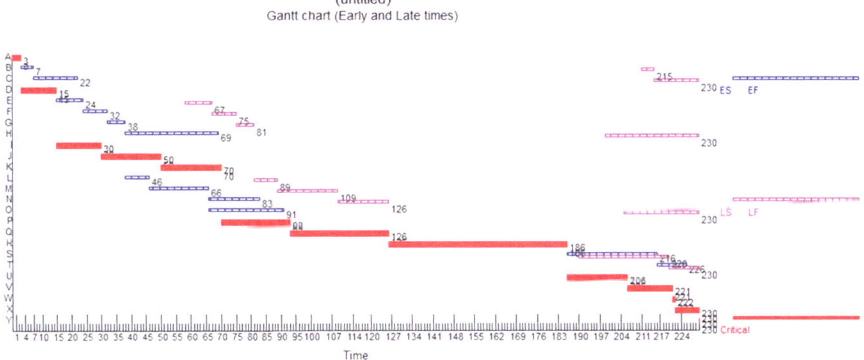

Fig. 14.8 Program Gantt chart

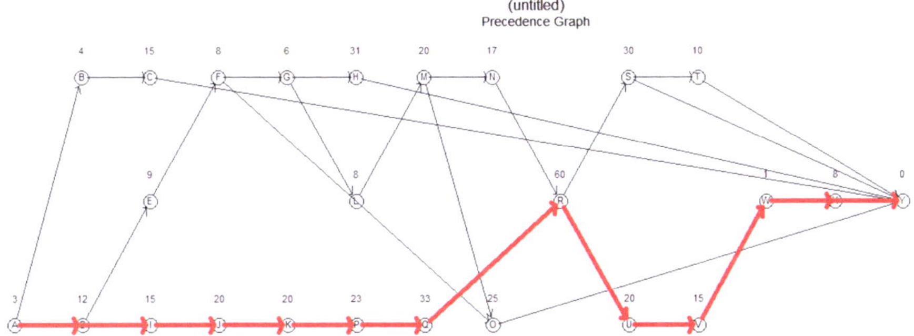

Fig. 14.9 PERT chart and table with critical path indicated

Activity	Activity time	Early Start	Early Finish	Late Start	Late Finish	Slack	Standard Deviation
Project	230						11.84
A	3	0	3	0	3	0	0.67
B	4	3	7	211	215	208	0.67
C	15	7	22	215	230	208	1.67
D	12	3	15	3	15	0	2.33
E	9	15	24	58	67	43	1.67
F	8	24	32	67	75	43	1.33
G	6	32	38	75	81	43	1.33
H	31	38	69	199	230	161	7.67
I	15	15	30	15	30	0	1.67
J	20	30	50	30	50	0	1.67
K	20	50	70	50	70	0	1.67
L	8	38	46	81	89	43	1.33
M	20	46	66	89	109	43	3.33
N	17	66	83	109	126	43	3.67
O	25	66	91	205	230	139	5
P	23	70	93	70	93	0	5
Q	33	93	126	93	126	0	9
R	60	126	186	126	186	0	0
S	30	186	216	190	220	4	3.33
T	10	216	226	220	230	4	1.67
U	20	186	206	186	206	0	2.67
V	15	206	221	206	221	0	3.33
W	1	221	222	221	222	0	0
X	8	222	230	222	230	0	1.33
Y	0	230	230	230	230	0	0

Fig. 14.9 (continued)

(EF), latest start (LS), and latest finish (EF) are the times that would be displayed in the box method for each activity.

For example, using activity L, advertise for lab assistants, node values would be:

L		8
38		46
81		89

Interpretation is that the earliest the advertising can start would be week 38 and is expected to take 8 weeks. The latest the advertisement could be placed is week 81 without the project running late. Therefore, there is a slack of 43 weeks.

For this example, we can see that the expected time to complete the research from beginning to publication is 230 days with a standard deviation of 11.84 days. This probabilistic approach is a beta distribution meaning that 50% of the time it can be completed before 230 days and 50% of the time it will be completed later than 230 days since the assumption is a normal distribution.

The red path designates the critical activities that must start and end on time to achieve the 230 days' finish time. If any activity on the critical path runs late, then the project will take longer than the expected time. This type of insight is the reason that PERT can be used as a tracking tool to confirm whether project tasks are on time or if there is a possibility of finishing ahead or behind the predicted time.

If the project schedule is running late, *crashing the project* can be considered. This is a technique used to bring the entire project back on schedule. When this happens, the activities on the critical path (and only ones on the critical path) are examined for the possibility of adding extra resources to bring the project back on track, usually at a monetary cost. However, there might be activities that are not amenable to timing adjustments. Therefore, you must identify the activities which cannot be shortened on the critical path. By putting extra resources on activities that *can* be shortened, a project can potentially be brought back on track. However, the critical path may have changed, and the PERT process will need to be recalculated [3].

14.4 Planning Budget and Project Expenses

A budget is a proposal that reflects the financials of the project. It is a list of anticipated costs that are the best estimate of what funds are needed to support the activities of a project during its proposed course of work. Creating a budget is important so that health scholars will understand the feasibility of their proposed project ideas. It is also a required item when seeking funds from a sponsoring organization.

Budgets are based on good faith estimates of the costs. Principles of good faith estimates include the cost being:

- Reasonable—a cost that would generally be accepted as necessary
- Necessary—a cost necessary to complete the project
- Allocable—a cost that can be allocated to a specific project in proportion to the benefits
- Allowable—a cost allowable according to guidelines

Health scholars need to think about what types of expenses the project will involve in order to outline budget categories that should be included in their project. Ideally, this list will include all items needed for a successful project.

The basic steps in determining a project's budget include the following:

- List the items necessary to accomplish the project
- Determine what the cost is reasonably going to be for each item

- Place the items in a spreadsheet
- Justify the items on the spreadsheet

Budget justification—an explanation and description of the types of individual costs that make up each larger budget category.

Sponsoring organizations often ask for details about how their funds will be used and provide budget forms. Common budget categories include:

- Personnel
- Employee benefits
- Supplies
- Travel
- Equipment
- Indirect costs

Budgets can be divided into fixed and variable costs. Other categories may be startup costs and in-kind (contribution/gift) donations. In an academic setting, the in-kind contributions may be in the form of classrooms, lab space, or personnel expertise such as a statistician's assistance. The value still must be acknowledged in the budget.

Many software programs are available for creating a budget and tracking project expenditures and costs. Templates can be edited to fit specific projects and will prompt consideration of categories that might otherwise have been overlooked. Once an acceptable spreadsheet is identified or modified, the budgeting task is simplified.

Costs can be cross-checked against the resource planning required. It is not uncommon to realize gaps after a careful review of the resource planning and budget. It is a good idea to return to the PERT chart after budgeting to make any necessary adjustments. A careful review of the project helps to fine-tune the project budget with the goal of not asking for too much or too little.

14.4.1 *Tracking Project Expenses*

Tracking expenses is important for several reasons. Expenses reveal the full range of support received by your organization or project. They also reflect the full range of resources you are managing as part of your project or the work of your organization. This may demonstrate that your project scope and capacity are greater than the cash-based budget alone would indicate. Tracking expenses is also how you keep your project within the budget.

The basic steps in tracking expenses include the following:

- Establish a cost tracking system.
- Set up parameters for what is permissible.
- Provide access to the tracking system.
- Assign someone to track the expenses

Tracking in-kind (donated) expenses warrants some additional caveats and explanations. In-kind donations are generally valued at their fair market rate or value at the time of donation. Valuations (the fair value) should be documented wherever possible.

- Space donations: The in-kind valuation in the case of donated space would be the fee charged as a space that is available for rental, based on established rental fee rates.
- Professional services: Free or pro bono services from licensed professionals should be valued at their existing rates for services.
- Volunteer time: Time by volunteers who are not professionals or specialists should not be valued at a rate that a professional would charge. For example, if a student handles your bulk mailing, their time should not be valued at the rate of a professional—the student would be considered a volunteer.
- Professional discounts: If you wish to value the difference between "market rate" and discounted rates agreed to by a vendor or colleague, keep in mind that the original rate should be documented (established).

It is preferable to keep and track in-kind valuations separate from tracking cash and instead show them as notes to the budget or within the project description. However, the value of in-kind donations is sometimes shown alongside the cash budget by creating a separate section in the budget spreadsheet. When in-kind valuations are shown as income on a budget balance sheet, then the budget *must* show the same amount as an expense on the balance sheet; this way, the amounts (and the budget) will balance.

14.5   Institutional Review

Institutions each have their own protocols and mechanisms for oversight. A health scholar must ensure that they carefully determine their own institution's requirements. If your project involves human subjects, it will require institutional review board (IRB) approval. The process of reviewing the application process requires thinking in-depth about the methodology, data collection, and analysis for the project. These tasks are part of the PERT analysis, and reevaluating the time and sequence may be considered. Statistics show that the average is 31 days for IRB approval, but approval can vary and take up to 6 months or longer.

14.6 Planning for Data Collection and Evaluation

It is important to consider the data collection at the beginning of a project to ensure that the appropriate information is collected in the right way to give the desired outcomes. Data collection techniques and evaluation must be thought through in detail to ensure that there is alignment in all aspects of the project. Even though the evaluation of the data might come after the execution of the project, all procedures for data collection and evaluation must be outlined in detail up front.

Questions to ask include the following:

- What type of data will be collected, quantitative or qualitative?
- What is the required sample size?
- What are the assumptions about the data, normal distribution or nonparametric?
- What statistical analysis/test will match the type of data, assumptions, and sample size?
- By whom and how will data be collected?
- Will data be collected and analyzed at the individual level or aggregated, and how will it be kept safe and anonymized?
- Is statistical software or qualitative software needed?
- What analysis method? Will a statistician be required?

Answers to these questions will feed into the resource planning, budget, PERT, logic model, and IRB application.

14.7 Resource Planning

Resource planning documents are categorized by materials, people, facilities, equipment, and software. Determining the people required can also be broken down further into administrative staff, professionals, laboratory staff, data specialists, etc. Continuing with more detail, describe the tasks for each person and needs as well as where do these tasks fall in the PERT chart.

The resource planning may point out:

- The necessity of scheduling a facility—the PERT chart might need revisiting
- Hiring staff with specific expertise—the budget might need revisiting
- Procuring equipment or software—the budget and PERT might need revisiting (Table 14.6)

Table 14.6 Resource requirement template

Resource needs	Activity/responsibility	Expense/cost
Human resources		
Administrative		
Professionals/educators		
Expertise		
Statistician		
Other		
Funding		
Grants		
In-kind		
Other support		
Facilities		
Office administrative		
Classroom		
Labs		
Other		
Materials		
Computers		
Educational textbooks		
Software		
Equipment/instrumentation		

14.8   Conclusion

Planning ahead takes effort, but the benefits of a well-thought-out plan far outweigh the investment and save time in the long run. Tools to consider using for initial organization are the logic model and high-level PERT as a project starting point. The logic model will help to make sure that gaps are not being forgotten. Following up with resource planning may point out missing steps such as recruitment of staff and scheduling facilities (classroom, labs, or ordering materials). Then the PERT chart can be updated. This iterative nature of the process is cumbersome but worthwhile so that major tasks and resources are included in planning. There are both free and paid versions of the templates available online. Using the tools and templates to plan and organize activities from the beginning of the project to the final publication submission will help the process proceed smoothly and result in fewer revisions and optimal use of time.

14.9 Questions

Discussion
1. When would you want to use:

    (a) A logic model
    (b) A Gantt chart
    (c) A PERT chart

Activities
1. Draft a logic model for your project.
2. Draft a resource requirements sheet for your project.

References

1. Issel LM, Wells R. Health program planning and evaluation. Jones and Bartlett, Burlington; 2018.
2. Malcolm DG, Roseboom JH, Clark CE, Fazar W. Application of a technique for research and development program evaluation. Oper Res. 1959;7(5):646–69.
3. Render B, Stair RM, Hanna ME. Quantitative analysis for management. Hoboken: Pearson/ Prentice Hall; 2009.

Further Reading

Bowerman B, O'Connell R, Murphree E. Business statistics and analytics in practice, 9th ed. McGraw-Hill Higher Education. 2019.
Timmereck T. Planning, program development, and evaluation. Burlington: Jones and Bartlett; 2003.
https://irb.uams.edu/2014/06/11/how-long-does-it-take-to-get-irb-approval-2/

Chapter 15
Support

Juliet M. Ray

15.1   Introduction

Seeking support for educational scholarship can seem like a daunting task and might even feel so intimidating that you might think it would be easier to do the project without anyone else's support. However, burnout is a significant problem for professionals and is even more acute among health professionals [1]. Ensuring that the proper resources are realizable is one of the most important actions a health scholar can take to ensure adequate support, their own well-being, and the success of a project.

There are different levels of support [2] with some levels requiring little planning and preparation and others requiring more time-intensive planning and preparation. In either case, there is basic information that will increase the likelihood of success. Steps include a realistic assessment of project needs, a clear understanding of sponsors and sponsored work, and a strategic plan to navigate the sponsored project landscape in ways that maximize successful project outcomes. This chapter outlines the process by breaking it down into component parts.

15.2   Decision to Seek Sponsorship

Whether or not to seek sponsored funding should be based fundamentally on the needs of the project. As described in prior chapters, determining project needs requires careful project planning. Funding considerations will require comparing the project's needs to the available resources and taking into consideration any

J. M. Ray (✉)
Johns Hopkins University School of Education, Baltimore, MD, USA
e-mail: jray29@jhu.edu

227

A. S. Fitzgerald, G. Bosch (eds.), *Education Scholarship in Healthcare*,
https://doi.org/10.1007/978-3-031-38534-6_15

institutional expectations for support. By performing such an analysis, a scholar can determine what support is needed for a successful project outcome. Such an analysis will also increase the chance of receiving support and help ensure compliance with organizational policies and procedures.

A health scholar will want to be strategic and consider future projects and career trajectory in addition to the immediate project at hand. This may look different depending on the professional setting but is worth considering. For example, starting with a smaller project, a limited budget, and seeking local funding is an excellent way to establish a good track record that builds credibility. The positive reputation then helps when later applying for larger or more prestigious awards. Another strategy is to collaborate with other scholars, especially senior scholars who may serve as mentors [3]. Being a member of another scholar's project team is a good way to learn about project management and the requirements of sponsors. This experience can later be highlighted in your resume as a signal to reviewers that you understand the process and are well equipped to lead your own project.

15.3　Project Planning

Previous chapters provided detailed information on what to consider in planning an educational scholarship project, including personnel, facilities, materials, equipment, instruments, and buy-in from stakeholders. Depending on the situation, these items might be available through your work, such as in-kind facilities' support or donations. But many times, outside funding is needed to make sure that the project has the resources needed to succeed. In either case, all expenses—whether they are directly charged to the project or not—should be included in the project plan to demonstrate the entire scope of the project. This detailed project planning is the first step to identifying the resources and associated costs needed to complete the project. You can use a logic model, PERT (Program Evaluation and Review Technique), or other planning tools as a starting point for resource planning and building the project budget.

There are several common categories of items to consider when associating cost with project requirements. These include personnel, travel, materials, consultants, and facilities and administration (F&A) costs (also known as indirect costs).

15.3.1　Personnel

Personnel costs are the funds needed for the people who are directly related to the project team. (Even though a consultant might be a team member, they are not "personnel" in this terminology.) During the planning phase, you will determine these costs by considering what expertise you will need on your team, identifying who has the expertise, and how much of each individual's time will be needed to complete the project.

Any individuals who will work on the project team and are from within your organization will likely be included under the heading of personnel costs unless there are extenuating circumstances (such as they are a hired consultant who is working at your workplace). Depending on the type of position or work agreement they hold with your institution, they might be paid hourly or through an annual salary, and your plan should reflect that status.

For personnel who receive an annual salary, consider what percentage of their time will be needed for the project, e.g., if they usually work 5 full days/week and you need them to work on the project for one full day each week, that is 20% effort. Effort can be any percentage 0–100% or in-kind (non-remuneration). This percentage can be multiplied by their annual salary. For hourly employees, consider how many hours it will take to do the project task. For both types of wages, there will likely be fringe benefits associated with their wage that will need to be accounted for in your budget. You can consult with the human resources department to find rate information that is specific to the organization. If your institution provides administrative staff to assist with research projects, they can also be helpful in this area and with budgeting more broadly.

15.3.2 Travel

Sometimes, travel is required to fulfill project activities. This might include mileage for the project team to visit sites or overnight travel to disseminate findings at professional conferences. Itemizing projected travel expenses demonstrates to reviewers that a project has been carefully planned. For example, budgeting mileage for team members to travel off-site in their personal car to collect data can be cost estimated using a reputable map source for distance calculation and an approved rate/distance to calculate the expense. Likewise, with overnight or alternate modes of travel, you will want to consult your organization's travel policies and use standard rates for lodging, airfare, train, and per diem (daily allowance for food or essentials).

15.3.3 Materials

The Materials category is broad and can include items ranging from online survey software to hardcopy paper and printing costs. An important distinction is between materials specific to the project (= Materials) and those that are simply basic office supplies (≠ Materials) as basic office supplies will usually fall under facilities and administration (F&A), below.

In the Materials category, it is important to be as detailed as possible. For most materials, it would be advisable to get a quote from a vendor who sells them. A quote should include the price per item, number of items needed, and any discounts. Providing a vendor quote as backup strengthens the justification of the funds requested in the Materials section of the plan.

15.3.4 Consultants

The Consultants category is for team members who are not employees of your organization/institution. Although some project teams are entirely composed of members from one organization, other teams have outside members to bring aspects of expertise or unique perspectives.

Payment arrangement to consultants varies by situation. You might hire a consultant to provide expertise in a specific area, needing them for a set amount of time and paying them hourly or a predetermined amount. An example of such a case would be the hiring of a statistician to assist with data analysis. To plan for a consulting statistician, you would determine the hourly rate a statistician charges, estimate the number of hours you would need for the project, and calculate the estimated cost. These calculations should be evident in the project plan.

In a different scenario, you might partner with several scholars from another institution who are responsible for a portion of the project. Under these circumstances, it is appropriate to consider issuing a subaward to the partner organization. Note that the subaward would be to the partner organization, not the individuals. Each organization/institution usually has requirements for creating subawards, including a detailed budget from the partner organization.

15.3.5 Facilities and Administrative Costs (or Indirect Costs)

The facilities costs that are included are those that support the project but are not easily identifiable [4]. Examples include the building, maintenance (janitorial, utilities, routine repairs), and library expenses. The administrative costs also support the project but again are not easily identifiable. Examples include accounting, payroll, and general administration.

15.4 Sponsored Support

Once you have identified the requirements of your project, you can look for sponsors. The process of identifying potential funding organizations is sometimes referred to as *prospect research* or *prospecting* [5]. Sponsors come from various avenues, but you will be looking for a match—a sponsor with similar goals and willing to provide the needed resources. Identifying the right sponsor requires due diligence and homework.

15.4.1 Where to Find Sponsors

There are several places to look for potential sponsors. Using an online search engine is a quick and easy first step. To make sure that you have identified the options at your institution, you might start with a search that has your institution and terms such as "small grant" to see what comes up. The next step would be to check your professional society web page for grant opportunities. Expanding the search terms to your local area plus terms such as philanthropy, grant, foundation, research funding, or "find a grant" will further identify potential funding organizations. Government agencies are in these funding databases, so it is advisable to also search within these agency websites.

If your institution has a research office, they might have access to funding databases that are behind paywalls. Some research offices send out funding opportunities regularly, and you can request to be added to their list of interested researchers who would like to receive information on any new opportunities (Table 15.1).

15.4.2 How to Find the Right Fit

There are several considerations when you look for a sponsor. First, consider whether the sponsor supports activities that share the same goals as your project [6]. Just as you consider an audience when deciding on a journal for publication or a

Table 15.1 Types of project sponsors

Support source	Intramural	Extramural			
Level	Programs at your institution	Local or regional	National private	National governmental	Global foundations
Example	Institution internal small grant program or faculty developmental award grant	Specialty organization small grant or local charitable foundation award	National medical society grant or a philanthropic organization grant	Government department with a mandate to further research in your area	Global organizations willing to support scholars

Consider starting with intramural support to build experience and reputation, and then apply for extramural support conference for poster presentation, so too do you consider the potential sponsor as an audience for your project. One way to learn about a potential sponsor is from their website. Pay attention to mission, vision, goals, and type of projects they have supported in the past. This first-level review is an opportunity to pare down lists, so time is not spent where a match is unlikely or undesirable.

Once you have a list that is workable in length (3–5 prospects), you can dive deeper into each sponsor to learn more about them. Many sponsor websites include a vast amount of information including organization annual reports, newsletters, and tax returns. This is valuable information. You can gain insight into what has been funded and how big/small the awards have been in the past. Then you can compare their previous awards to your project planning estimate of needs to make sure that each potential sponsor can support your project at the level needed to be successful. If the support level available is below your estimate of need but you still want to apply to them for sponsorship, you might consider breaking your project into discrete sections that could be funded in smaller parts, a process known as *chunking*.

Most funding organizations provide eligibility requirements to make it clear who may apply. This can include specifics such as membership in a specific society or career timing, e.g., early-career scholars or 5–10 years after training. This can be a benefit to you if you fit the criteria as it limits the pool of potential applicants. At the same time, if you do not fit the criteria, do not waste time working on a proposal for which you cannot be awarded.

It is advisable to narrow your list down to two or three strong prospects and then take the next step to reach out to the sponsor. It is recommended to create a one-page summary of your project idea that can be shared with potential sponsors when making contact. Some sponsors will list a point of contact such as a program officer on their website. This is the person who can answer questions about the sponsor and the specific grant program. The one-page summary can be sent to the contact along with a note asking if it would be possible to schedule a brief call/meeting.

The one-page preview of your overall project plan will increase the efficiency of subsequent contact with the potential sponsor. You need to prepare for the call/meeting by making a list of questions you want to ask them. Be prepared to take notes.

If a potential sponsor does not post a point of contact or program officer on their website, you might consider checking within your organization to see if a relationship with the sponsor already exists. If so, a point of contact or introduction might be possible.

15.5   Organizational/Institutional Requirements

Each organization (institution) usually has policies and guidelines for how grants are handled to ensure compliance with best practices. It is helpful to seek out the staff in the office that is responsible for grant compliance and ask for their assistance. They can often aid with the process of finding funding and ensure that you are following the relevant policies. At an institution of higher education, the office might have a title such as Office of Sponsored Projects/Programs.

Some of the typical services provided by such an office are (1) assistance in finding appropriate funding opportunities, (2) networking with other scholars interested in the same area of research, and (3) assistance with budgeting. Budgeting assistance is particularly important since the staff would have insight into up-to-date information on fringe benefit rates and F&A rates for the organization. The staff might also have budget templates tailored specifically to your organization. Other types of support include access to organizational templates and (less commonly) grant writing assistance.

15.5.1 Organizational Compliance

Many organizational compliance policies require projects to seek approval before they begin, so health scholars should be aware of the compliance regulations that might impact their projects. Specific policies are subject to change over time and might differ by region. Often, there are staff within organizations who specialize in these areas and can provide up-to-date guidance and support for compliance.

Common compliance issues include the following:

- Effort reporting—how personnel time is accounted for must be tracked and reported
- Institutional review board—for the protection of human subjects
- Institutional Animal Care and Use Committee—for the protection of animal subjects
- Conflict of interest and/or commitment—to protect research integrity

15.6 Sponsored Projects

A *sponsored project* is a research, service, or instructional project that is supported by an entity outside the institution (the sponsor), based on a commitment where terms are agreed upon by both parties, and the sponsor receives a benefit [7].

A sponsored project binds an institution to a specific line of scholarly inquiry, and the sponsor may maintain control over the project direction, oversight, and administration. Different sponsors require differing levels of control and involvement in the project. These issues are addressed by different types of agreements and are specified in the terms and conditions. These agreements are often a result of a request for proposal (RFP) that has been released by the sponsor and the submission of a proposal to the RFP that has been made by the research team.

By contrast, gifted funds can have stipulations but no expectation of benefit to the sponsor. The distinction between gifts, grants, and sponsored projects is important to institutions, so a health scholar might need to consult with their institution's research office if their situation is ambiguous.

15.7 Proposal Development

After identifying the project requirement, narrowing the potential sponsors to a few well-matched in fit, checking with your organization for their requirements, and understanding the type of sponsorship you are seeking (sponsored project or gift), the next step is to develop a proposal. To be successful, you must clearly understand the sponsor's expectations for the proposal. Most sponsors have detailed guidelines to follow, while others are informal. To gain clarity, it is imperative to read any provided guidelines closely for guidance on information to include or exclude. Note whether any specific headings and subheadings are required for the various sections of the proposal. Even font size, line spacing, and margins are often noted. These details may sound minor, but they are asking for uniformity in appearance, so reviewers can better judge content. Proposals are often administratively returned without review for failure to adhere to guidelines. Writing a proposal is hours of work, and no one wants to be turned down because of the font.

As you study the sponsor's submission guidelines, it is helpful to create a proposal checklist. On the list, include each required document or task, when you need it completed, and who will be responsible for bringing the document/task to completion. If you have a project team, this is a good time to practice your teambuilding by allowing others to play active roles with the responsibility to help in the process. Also, consult with any organizational research office or administration staff who might be able to offer expert tips and timeline suggestions. Organizations often have internal routing requirements and approval processes that need to be completed before your final submission to the sponsor, so an additional margin for timing should be built in to allow for this step. Table 15.2 lists the most common components and provides a brief description.

Table 15.2 Common components of a proposal

Proposal element	Description
Letter of intent, if applicable	Outline of project activities, amount requested, and basic demographic information on the project team
Cover page	Demographic and administrative information for organization and project team
Statement of need	Description of the problem, target population, impact of the project
Project narrative	Project objectives, methodology, outcomes
References	Sources cited
Budget	An itemized list of project expenses
Budget justification	A narrative description of the purpose and need of budgeted items
Project team description	Description of experience and expertise of project team—can include biosketches, resumes, or curriculum vitae

15.8 Proposal Review and Submission

Once you have completed the full proposal package, it is a good idea to go back and review it before submission. There are several types of review, and which one you choose will likely depend on the size and scope of the project.

Self-review. This review includes copy editing to check readability and ensure that all grammar and punctuation are correct. Reviewers are not always experts in your field, so make sure that you use clear language and avoid academic jargon. In this step, look back at the guidelines and compare them to your proposal. Check to make sure that the proposal meets *all* of the sponsor requirements. Some guidelines include evaluation criteria. This can be a valuable resource. Use it to review your proposal, and check that you have included all the components so you have the greatest chance of success.

Peer review. Ask a colleague to review your proposal. Your peer can provide copy editing but usually does not provide an administrative review of guidelines. Peer review is valuable for improving readability. Even someone who is not familiar with your field can provide valuable feedback on how clearly you presented your ideas in layman's terms.

Mentor review. A mentor's review of your proposal can provide valuable feedback from their own proposal experiences. Plan ahead by asking the mentor early in your process about their willingness to help review, and then give them dates for when you plan to provide a draft and when you will need their feedback to meet the submission deadline. Allow ample time for the mentor to review and ask questions if their suggestions are unclear in substance or reason.

Panel review. This option is generally only used with very large, multidisciplinary proposals. This is an effective but time-consuming review so reserved for cases that involve significant funding. Multiple individuals simulate the proposal review panel by evaluating the proposal in depth using the sponsor's criteria and then providing feedback to the author.

Institutional review and approval. The final approval is required before a proposal can be submitted through an organization. The steps differ by institution but usually take the form of multiple individuals reviewing a proposal to make sure that all budgetary and administrative requirements are met.

Sponsor review (upon submission). The sponsor will review the proposal, and you will receive an evaluation (scoring, rating, feedback) with meaningful insights. If not accepted, take any scoring or feedback into consideration when revising the proposal, and resubmit at the next opportunity. It is not uncommon for projects to be awarded on a second or third attempt, so do not see an initial rejection as failure; instead, see resubmissions as increasing the chance of success (if you have appropriately revised your proposal).

15.9   Stewardship of Funding Support

Stewardship is the job of taking care of the award for support. A health scholar must understand the responsibilities that come along with receiving external support for a project. Sponsors usually ask for reports as a condition of their award, but even if they do not, providing updates in 6- to 12-month intervals is a part of good stewardship and will build credibility and rapport with the sponsor. Stewardship reports fall into two main categories, programmatic reporting and financial reporting. It will be the health scholar's responsibility to track when these reports are due and remind any team members of upcoming deadlines.

At the time of a sponsorship award, the health scholar should call a meeting of the project team. It is particularly important to have present at the meeting any team members who will be responsible for major tasks or tracking finances.

At the meeting:

- Review the project proposal in detail as it was approved by the sponsor
- Ensure that there is a common understanding of what must be done and who is responsible
- Review the project timeline from start to completion
- Review the budget paying particular attention to adjustments made as part of the award process

15.9.1   Programmatic Reporting

The programmatic report tells sponsors how the project is progressing toward meeting its goals and objectives. At the time of award, sponsors usually provide detailed guidelines for how this information should be presented and at what intervals. Details of the report usually include a comparison of the project's current progress toward the goals compared to the timeline originally given in the proposal and an estimation of time to project completion. Specific information in the report is unique to each project but might include details such as participant recruitment efforts, data collection and analysis, or deliverables.

15.9.2   Financial Reporting

Financial bookkeeping requires checks and balances with documentation and fiscal controls. The official award budget will be included in your award agreement. Ensure that all team members are aware of the award budget (which might differ from the proposal budget) and that only the official award budget is used as the basis for financial reporting.

Basic financial stewardship rules include the following:

- Create a system for organizing and tracking finances, including expenditures, receipts, and other documentation
- Monitor spending, and reconcile to project budget regularly (monthly, quarterly, yearly)
- Have checks and balances in place that involve more than one person
- Only allow expenses that are in the approved budget and for the approved purpose
- Contact the sponsor for approval if a change to the budget is needed

Good financial stewardship practices help keep a project on budget. Your institution may be able to offer assistance with the financial tracking of funds. The institutional resources can help you meet the award requirements and also support compliance with institutional policies, but it will be the health scholar's responsibility to ensure that good stewardship practices are followed for the project.

15.10 Conclusion

External support can be a crucial component of a successful educational scholarship project. Generating support and assembling the required resources up front increase the likelihood that a project will successfully meet its goals. While it can be tempting to shortcut these early steps in hopes to get by with what is on hand, new scholars often underestimate the time and funding needed to complete tasks. As outlined in previous chapters, projects are multidimensional and do not always adhere to a schedule. Delays and challenges occur. Preplanning and engaging with external funding organizations strengthen a health scholar's credentials. More resources allow for variances in projects while also increasing the professional network and can increase the net impact of the final product. The right sponsor fit is a win-win situation for both the health scholar and the sponsor.

15.11 Questions

Discussion Questions
1. Do you see any opportunities to obtain internal support from your department, division, or institution?
2. Where can you find resources to locate external funding sources?
3. What are your thoughts on seeking funding from private or commercial sources?

Activities
1. Make a list of potential internal and external funding sources for your project.

References

1. Morgantini LA, Naha U, Wang H, Francavilla S, Acar Ö, Flores JM, et al. Factors contributing to healthcare professional burnout during the COVID-19 pandemic: a rapid turnaround global survey. PLoS One. 2020;15(9):e0238217. https://doi.org/10.1371/journal.pone.0238217.
2. Smith N, Tremore J. The everything grant writing book. 2nd ed. Avon: Adams Media; 2008.
3. Moore JB. Choosing an academic team and being a team player: part I. In: JPHMP direct: a companion site to the Journal of Public Health Management and Practice. 2018. https://jphmpdirect.com/2018/05/04/choosing-an-academic-team-and-being-a-team-player-part-i/. Accessed 26 Mar 2022.
4. 2 CFR§200.56 Indirect (facilities and administrative (F&A)) costs.
5. Greater Public. Grant seekers toolkit step 2: prospect research. 2022. https://greaterpublic.org/resources/major-planned-giving/grant-seekers-toolkit-step-2-prospect-research/. Accessed 26 Mar 2022.
6. Moore JB. Grant writing in academic public health—the basics. In: JPHMP direct: a companion site to the Journal of Public Health Management and Practice. 2019. https://jphmpdirect.com/2019/04/05/grant-writing-in-academic-public-health-the-basics/. Accessed 26 Mar 2022.
7. Johns Hopkins University School of Nursing (JHU SON). Sponsored research handbook. 2020. https://nursing.jhu.edu/faculty_research/research/sponsored-projects/documents/SponsoredHandbook.pdf. Accessed 26 Mar 2022.

Chapter 16
Mentors, Coaches, and Facilitators

Patricia A. Thomas and Anne E. Belcher

16.1   Introduction

A 1977 qualitative study of 72 American Nobel laureates found that the single most important key to their success was the mentor [1]. Fifty-eight percent of these Nobel Prize winners were taught or mentored by Nobel Prize winners—an enduring phenomenon now referred to as the "family tree" of Nobel laureates.

Having an effective mentoring relationship is one of the most powerful tools in the health scholar's toolbox as well. Academic mentors, by virtue of their expertise and experience, promote the personal and professional development of mentees and are particularly useful in guiding younger colleagues through both the explicit and implicit rules of academic life. Mentoring predicts improved research productivity, success in promotion and tenure, and career and job satisfaction [2–8]. Mentoring is now a core competency in the Nursing Professional Development Scope and Standards of Practice [9]. The mentor is so important to the research enterprise that it has become a criterion of select funding programs, such as the NIH Research Career Development (K) awards, the Veterans Affairs Career Development Awards, and the Macy Faculty Scholars Program.

The presence of the mentor helps the busy clinician educator to overcome several barriers to scholarship, such as trying to balance work and personal life, completing clinical demands, and time-consuming assignments distributed by attending staff. The most common uses of mentors for clinician educators are career guidance and

P. A. Thomas (✉)
Department of Medicine, Johns Hopkins University School of Medicine,
Baltimore, MD, USA
e-mail: pathomas@jhmi.edu

A. E. Belcher
Johns Hopkins University School of Education, Baltimore, MD, USA
e-mail: abelche2@jhu.edu

A. S. Fitzgerald, G. Bosch (eds.), *Education Scholarship in Healthcare*,
https://doi.org/10.1007/978-3-031-38534-6_16

emotional support [10]. The mentor can also guide the mentee in a specific educational project, set timelines and accountability targets, teach writing skills, provide critical feedback and encouragement when needed, and gradually build the mentee's professional self-esteem and self-confidence [11].

With the increased complexity of faculty roles, it is difficult for a single mentor to meet all the expectations of these relationships. Less than 50%, and in some studies 20%, of faculty report having a mentor, and the availability and feasibility of experienced mentors are frequent barriers to mentoring programs [11]. The lack of mentors is one of five identified barriers to scholarship across multiple health professions [12]. The most at-risk faculty seem least likely to be mentored. Studies consistently report that fewer women faculty have identified mentors [7, 8, 13, 14], and some worry that the current environment may worsen these numbers [15]. Underrepresented minority faculty experience lower career satisfaction, coupled with feelings of alienation and seclusion, and have lower success in academic promotion and tenure, yet receive less frequent mentorship [16–18]. To address these issues, new forms and models of mentoring are evolving, such as *functional mentoring* and *peer mentors*, and the use of *coaches* in professional development.

This chapter contrasts the academic mentor and coach relationships, explores the benefits and risks of both, and presents what is known about best practices for success. A description of alternative models of faculty mentorship and what is known about their effectiveness follows. The chapter concludes with thoughts on other facilitators for career success.

16.2 Mentors and Coaches

Since the mentor role is as old as human history, most of us have a working definition of a mentor, although dozens of definitions have been published. Briefly, a mentor is a trusted counselor or guide. The credibility and authority of the mentor come from age, experience, and recognized expertise in the field. In academia, the traditional model of the mentor is best exemplified by the research mentor-mentee dyad. When a junior researcher joins a research lab or center, the director of the lab/center assumes the role of mentor, teaching procedures and techniques, guiding research focus, providing resources, co-authoring publications, and facilitating networking. As the work supervisor, the mentor is physically available and provides performance feedback over a longitudinal relationship. Good mentors are described as altruistic and active listeners and generously provide knowledge of the organization and profession. Successful mentees eventually become independent investigators and go on to establish their research labs/centers, at which point the formal relationship ends and is replaced by collegial interactions that can continue for years.

Clinical and educator faculty can also serve as mentors to health scholars, although it is less common to see as intense a relationship as that described above. Mentoring for career development is usually a long-term commitment; a relationship may begin at the time of postgraduate training or faculty recruitment and continue for years into the faculty appointment. More commonly, a mentor agrees to assist with the development, implementation, and dissemination of an educational project, with a shorter timeline. As with researchers, senior clinical faculty can adopt many roles in a mentoring relationship: serve as professional role models; teach the balance of multiple academic roles; guide time management; advise clinical productivity; advocate and sponsor faculty in professional networking; deliver constructive feedback in scholarly writing; and provide accountability or encouragement when needed.

Coaching is a newer model of career development and facilitation in academia. Coaching often refers to performance improvement but can be focused on deeper cognitive or psychological issues. Carmel and Paul have defined coaching as "a helping relationship between (a) a less experienced academic (acting as a client) and (b) a more experienced academic (acting as a consultant) who uses a range of behavioral and other techniques to help the less experienced academic achieve a mutually identified set of goals, agreed upon formally or informally. In this relationship, a coach facilitates a client's active engagement, learning, and commitment to a course of action" [19]. Coaching assumes that the client has strengths and skills that are not being accessed effectively [20].

The principles of coaching hold across disciplines [21]. The relationship is forged with active listening to build connections between coach and client. There is usually an assessment phase, in which the client self-assesses strengths and areas of needed development, often using checklists or instruments. Inquiry is used to guide client insight. The client next sets a specific measurable goal to be achieved, and the coach elicits a commitment to that goal. An action plan is generated. The last phase is continuous assessment and support as the client works through the action plan.

Two uses of the coaching model have been for longitudinal advising relationships in postgraduate training and for addressing specific performance issues, such as communication issues with patients or colleagues, or ethical lapses in prescribing patterns. In the longitudinal model, the assigned coach may work with the trainee over several years, and it is important to have a formalized structure that details the frequency of meetings, topics to be addressed, and methods of communication. For the latter use of performance improvement, the relationship may be structured to end when the coach and client agree that the performance skill has been achieved.

Mentor and coach mentoring dyads are similar in that both begin with a values clarification exercise so that both parties understand the goals of the mentee (values clarification exercises help one to increase their awareness of any values that may impact lifestyle decisions and actions; exercises may include reflection, completing a values assessment tool, and sorting and prioritizing named values, or the coach/mentor may be actively involved in using inquiry to elicit and rank values) [22]. As noted, both mentor and coach relationships may use written agreements to confirm the structure, commitment, and goals of the relationship, i.e., the professional and personal development of the mentee. The mentor and coach share the need to create a safe environment for the mentee that encourages trust, uses active listening, provides emotional support and encouragement, and serves as a professional role model.

Mentors and coaches differ, however, in important ways. Whereas mentors have unique seniority and expertise in the field, the coach may not even be in the same discipline. Mentors are expected to provide access to resources, networking, and advocacy and to create opportunities for the mentee to advance in the field. The coach's role is to encourage the client to use their own acknowledged strengths, to focus on personal areas in need of improvement, and to develop reflexivity (the habit of critical reflection on one's actions) as a skill for lifelong career development. Advice may pop up in coaching sessions, but the experienced coach should quickly check in with the client to ensure that the client is doing the active work of problem-solving.

16.3 The Mentor-Mentee Dyad Relationship

16.3.1 Finding and Initiating a Mentoring Relationship

Some organizations have recognized the critical value of mentoring/coaching for those entering a profession and have formalized programs that support this activity for both participants. Such programs prepare the senior mentor/coach for the role, facilitating the success of the relationship. If there is no formalized mechanism for a junior health scholar to be matched with a mentor/coach, the responsibility of securing the mentor falls to the junior. Lack of support for the senior faculty member to serve as a mentor can be a significant barrier for those trying to identify mentors. Most senior faculty are flattered, if not honored, to be asked to serve as mentors, regardless of funding or organizational support. Nevertheless, the junior faculty member needs to understand that the mentor may be juggling multiple commitments and unable to provide the access that feeds an effective mentoring relationship.

Both trainees and faculty report that the most successful mentor-mentee relationships are those that have been selected by the mentee [6, 23, 24]. The Nobel laureates interviewed in 1977 had chosen their mentors before they had received a Nobel laureate, indicating that they were particularly perceptive about their mentorship. In identifying a mentor, the junior faculty member may be drawn to one with prestige, or a particularly charismatic teacher/clinician. The literature frequently lists ideal mentor characteristics that may read like an application for sainthood [25] (see Table 16.1). What seems to be most important in successful mentoring, however, is the quality of the interactions between the mentor and mentee. Optimal mentoring involves several interactional foundations: mentee-centeredness, emotional safety, support, informality, responsiveness, and respect [26]. Having a personal rapport may be more important than the seniority of the mentor [13]; in fact, age differences can hinder the relationship [27]. Key characteristics of successful mentoring relationships are mutual respect, personal connection, and shared values [10].

Table 16.1 Characteristics and behaviors of good mentors

- Altruistic, selfless, generous
- Emotionally intelligent
- Invested in and committed to mentee's success
- Available, flexible, accessible, reliable
- Demonstrable honesty, integrity, and trustworthiness
- Significant mentor experience
- Knowledge of the organization, professional field, and academic culture
- Active listener
- Engagement in self-reflection
- Advisement of mentee on setting and attaining career goals
- Recognition of mentee's strengths and areas in need of development
- Identification of clinical and scholarly opportunities for the mentee
- Assistance with professional networking
- Provision of challenges and accountability as needed
- Provision of constructive and practical feedback
- Creation of a safe environment, assurance of confidentiality
- Provision of emotional support
- Sensitivity to work-life balance issues
- Responsiveness to issues associated with gender, race/ethnicity, lifestyle, and class
- Advocacy for scholarship and academic integrity

[a] Adapted from Haines [4], Straus [10], Carmel and Paul [19], Geraci and Thigpen [25]

If you are planning to ask for mentorship, you need to do an honest and critical self-evaluation before making the request (see Table 16.2). This should result in the ability to articulate your short- and long-term career goals, current priorities, and expectations of what mentorship can provide at this point. Once you have clarified what you need, you can start the process of identifying one or more mentors that meet that need.

Early in the faculty appointment, it is most helpful to have someone in the same organization who understands the organizational culture and helps you to integrate successfully into that culture [28]. Gender and race/ethnicity concordance is helpful, but not critical and often not available in more senior faculty. Work supervisors are not considered ideal mentors as they may be conflicted concerning one's time management, career focus, and performance feedback. Asking supervisors or peers for recommendations can help to identify good mentors. Think broadly—your ideal mentor may be in a different department or organizational unit. Meet with people to seek advice. Once you have identified a potential mentor, ask for a meeting, and be specific with your request, based on your self-evaluation. Difficulty in scheduling a meeting may be a red flag that the potential mentor is already overcommitted.

Table 16.2 Managing a mentoring relationship

Stage	Components	Comments
• *Prepare*		
	Perform a Critical Self-Evaluation:	
	What are your short-term (1–3 years) and long-term (5–10 years) career goals?	
	What are your perceived barriers in achieving these goals?	
	What do you see as your strengths/unique attributes in achieving these goals?	
	Are there gaps in knowledge or skills that need additional training/practice?	
	How could a mentor assist you in achieving these goals?	
	What are your current work-life priorities?	
	What are you struggling with currently in your clinical practice, teaching, scholarly productivity, and personal relationships?	
	How do you respond to feedback?	
	How do you respond to professional challenges?	
	How much time could you commit to a mentoring relationship now?	
	Are you willing and able to accept responsibility for managing the mentoring relationship?	
• *Identify a mentor*		
	Look for someone you respect because of role modeling, professional expertise, shared professional interests, interpersonal skills, and scholarly productivity	
	Ask supervisors or colleagues to suggest potential mentors	
	Think broadly across the institution for potential mentors	
	Meet with individuals to explore interests, shared values, and personal rapport	
	Approach the invitation with respect and clarity about your expectations	
• *Cultivate and sustain the relationship*		
	State your expectations and hoped-for outcomes	
	Negotiate the frequency of meetings and frequency and method of communications	
	Use project plans or timelines as structure	
	Arrive for meetings on time and well prepared	
	Communicate respectfully	
	Be honest about challenges	
	Summarize meetings and next steps	
	Express gratitude	
	Periodically assess the quality of the relationship: complete the Mentorship Effectiveness Scale and ask the mentor how it is going from their perspective	
• *Transitions*		
	Anticipate termination	
	Reflect on what has been accomplished	
	Share what has been learned and the impact of the relationship on both	
	Express gratitude and seek advice for next steps	

[a] Adapted from Haines [4], Zerzan [29], Carey and Weissman [11], Straus [10]

The first meeting is a key opportunity to "manage up the relationship" [29]—arrive on time, acknowledge and thank the mentor, present an organized agenda for the meeting, communicate your goals, and negotiate optimum timing and communications for future meetings. After the meeting, send a brief email expressing thanks, summarizing the meeting, and suggesting an agenda for the next meeting. These activities demonstrate respect, your active listening and receptivity to the mentor's input and schedule, and your willingness to assume responsibility for the relationship.

16.3.2 Maximizing the Mentor-Mentee Relationship

Unless required by a formal program or funding organization, it is unusual to have formal written agreements between academic mentors and mentees. The relationship may be fostered, however, by including a discussion of the mutual responsibilities and expectations up front. Table 16.3 shows an example of a project timeline for a publication that can form the basis of a discussion with the mentor.

Plan how you can best use the time spent with the mentor and how you are contributing to the relationship over time. Show up for meetings on time. Have a specific agenda for meetings. If you have received feedback, reflect on your application of that feedback at the next meeting. If you are working on scholarship, meet agreed-upon short-term goals or tasks for the next meeting. Be open and honest with the challenges you are facing.

Successful mentor-mentee relationships are mutually beneficial. For mentors, the frequent meaningful interactions with the mentee result in greater productivity,

Table 16.3 Setting a project timeline for a scholarly publication

Task	Mentee	Target date	Mentor	Target date
Clarify aims and goals				
Identify collaborators and authors				
Complete background literature search				
Submit IRB application				
Collect data and complete analysis				
Select journal and review author instructions				
Assign paper sections to authors				
Assemble first draft				
Check references and formatting				
Confirm author order				
Submit to journal				
Respond to reviewers' comments				
Review proofs				
Plan for dissemination (visual abstract, social media, etc.)				

career satisfaction, and personal gratification in working with effective mentees [30]. The mentee experiences transformative learning and growth in professional identity [4]. Mentoring relationships can be complicated, however, by personality mismatch, poor communication styles, wavering commitment, and even competition [10]. Periodically, check in with yourself and the mentor regarding the effectiveness of the relationship. Berk's "Mentoring Effectiveness Checklist" is a helpful tool for this conversation [31].

### 16.3.3	Transitions

It is natural that over time (generally 2–5 years), the needs of the mentee change, and a re-evaluation of the relationship is in order. The mentee may seek more autonomy and independence, and this phase of the relationship may lead to a decision to separate. As with the other phases of the relationship, this should be managed explicitly and respectfully, discussing the optimal timing of separation, and seeking advice for the next steps in the mentee's career. Done well, the mentor-mentee relationship transitions to a lifelong friendship and collegial relationship.

## 16.4	Other Models of Mentorship

Regardless of which model one is using, the mentee's activities should reflect those described above: begin with a reflective values clarification, accept responsibility for the relationship, approach with respect, and honor the time of all individuals.

In the absence of supportive organizations, there may be limited senior faculty available for the mentor-mentee dyad described above. There are, however, multiple opportunities for mentorship and willing mentors. *Informal mentors* embed mentoring activities in their daily work, sharing knowledge and skills with less experienced colleagues, or checking in with new colleagues to provide encouragement and emotional support. Nearly every health professional has experienced working with a *preceptor* in a particular clinical setting, who provides guidance and feedback to the trainee over a defined period, which is an example of informal mentoring.

### 16.4.1	Functional Mentors

Whereas the traditional model focuses on the compatibility of mentor and mentee in a reciprocal relationship, the functional model focuses on the mentor having needed skills and knowledge for a particular project. Functional mentors may provide feedback on teaching a particular course, advice on preparing a grant submission, guidance on completion of a scholarly project, or tips on setting up a clinical practice.

The mentor is one who has modeled professionalism and success and agrees to share knowledge and skills for the duration of the "function." Similarly, functional mentors may be identified for career advice or managing work-life balance. When project based, the outcomes of a successful functional mentoring relationship directly benefit the organization [30]. Functional mentors are often available through professional societies and faculty development programs [32].

16.4.2 Peer Mentors

Peer mentors are at the same career level who agree to provide information and feedback to each other, often alternating the mentor role and building their mentoring skills. Closer to the experience and issues being faced, peers may be more empathic with one experiencing career challenges. Collegial peers are collaborators on a scholarly project that agree to engage in constructive feedback and share resources for the project. Disadvantages of the peer model are the potential for more competition between the parties and the lack of expert input when misinformation or missteps arise [11].

16.4.3 Facilitated Peer Groups

To address these issues, a structured model of *facilitated peer groups* has emerged. This allows the accommodation of several mentees, all of whom have access to relevant information and skill-building. These programs often include a values clarification exercise, opportunities to validate each participant's goals and struggles, and completion of faculty development workshops centered on career development and scholarship. The program may also include the completion of a joint scholarly project that generates opportunities to build knowledge and skills. One program has demonstrated that faculty emerge from such a longitudinal program with identification of core values, structured career planning, skill development in negotiation, conflict management, scholarly writing, and development of collaborative relationships in the workplace [33].

16.4.4 Network and Multiple Mentors

Distance, virtual, and telementoring have recently emerged as approaches to mentoring when local resources are insufficient, or mentors and mentees are geographically separated [7, 34].

It is the natural history of a faculty career to accrue a *network of mentors* that may include senior faculty, leaders, peers, and other colleagues. Each relationship may sustain a different aspect of one's professional and personal development and together create a mentoring community for the participant. This is also referred to as the *mosaic model* of mentoring. While this avoids reliance on a single mentor, one disadvantage is the lack of "big picture" oversight of one's activities [11]. One study concluded that mentors from professional societies were the most helpful to faculty, while local institutional mentors were the least helpful [35].

16.5 Becoming a Mentor

With experience, the health scholar accumulates the knowledge and skills to be a mentor. For many, this role is embedded in the profession, and it is an expectation that one assumes the role of teacher and guide to the junior professional. For others, the opportunity to shape professional identities and nurture the junior professional is a privilege. Perhaps, the most important consideration before stepping into this role is to honestly assess whether you have the time and capacity to take on the role of mentor, remembering that accessibility and responsiveness are key to effective mentoring.

Once again, a critical self-assessment may help you to develop as an effective mentor. What strengths do you have as a mentor? What challenges do you see in serving as a mentor? Do you have the time to commit to a mentoring relationship? What feedback could your mentee provide you along the way? How will you judge the success of the relationship?

If you are committed to assuming this role, explore opportunities to develop mentoring skills through your professional society or other faculty development programs. Deepen your knowledge of adult learners and millennial learners. Reflect on professional boundaries encountered in mentoring relationships. Learn and practice skills of active listening, giving constructive feedback, responding to microaggressions, communicating with empathy, and recognizing when someone is in trouble. Seek out other experienced mentors as coaches as you embark on this new role and anticipate the need to seek mentorship for mentoring.

16.6 Other Facilitators to Career Success

As noted above, there is increasing organizational awareness of the importance of mentoring to facilitate recruitment and retention of talented health professions scholars, and there are many efforts to build a "culture of mentoring." Departments have launched programs to facilitate matching with a mentor, using mentee-initiated, speed-dating with mentors, or guided matching—gender, race, lifestyle, and family status—which have been shown to facilitate success. Providing faculty development for building mentoring skills, supporting protected time, identifying resources to monitor and evaluate mentoring, including mentoring plans in hiring procedures, and celebrating successful mentoring all contribute to the culture of mentoring [36]. Mentoring academies are another approach to facilitate the process of matching new employees with experienced mentors; many have engaged professional alumni to serve as mentors and coaches. Teaching and mentoring academies may offer faculty development workshops in mentoring skills and writing for publication. These same academies may also sponsor competitive *grants for educational projects.*

Awards for mentoring excellence are now common in professional schools. Some schools also include consideration of mentoring activity in promotion decisions or provide financial supplements for department heads that have developed robust mentoring programs. Institutional incentives for mentoring are associated with mentors' perception of the benefits of mentoring [37].

Longitudinal faculty development programs (such as the Macy Faculty Scholars and the Harvard Macy Program for Educators), *post-residency educational fellowships, and masters' degree programs in health professions education*, if feasible, are particularly effective in developing a health scholar's career [38, 39]. Most include content dedicated to curriculum development, teaching skills, adult learning theory, and educational scholarship and require the completion of a thesis/scholarly project. Participants in these longitudinal experiences engage with mentors and peers who enrich a mentoring community long after the end of the program.

Most professional societies and hospitals sponsor *leadership development programs* or *tracks*, offering training and development in leadership skills that can facilitate promotion to new roles, and result in career advancement for the health scholar.

16.7 Conclusion

Mentoring in academia describes an intentional reciprocal relationship between a more experienced mentor and a less experienced mentee, to promote the mentee's professional development and career success. Successful relationships are grounded in shared values, good communication, personal rapport, and mutual respect. Choosing the right mentor and managing the relationship are increasingly the responsibility of the mentee. New models and technologies are evolving to meet the needs of junior faculty.

16.8 Questions

Discussion Questions
1. Do you have a culture of mentorship in your current professional environment? If not, what would you need to change to establish such an environment?
2. In your opinion or in your experience, what characteristics are needed by an effective mentor for meaningful educational or scholarly work?

Activities

1. List the mentor qualities that you feel are important for effective collaboration.
2. List the personal barriers you anticipate to accomplishing your project, drafting your manuscript, and ensuring the publication of your work.
3. Who are potential mentors with both the qualities listed in your response to #1 above *and* the ability to help you overcome the personal barriers you listed in #2 above?

*Hint: The right mentor may or may not be more senior and may or may not have a prestigious title.

References

1. Zuckerman H. Scientific elite: Nobel laureates in the United States. 2nd ed. New York: Routledge; 2017.
2. DeCastro R, Griffith KA, Ubel PA, Stewart A, Jagsi R. Mentoring and the career satisfaction of male and female academic medical faculty. Acad Med. 2014;89(2):301–11.
3. Hafsteinsdóttir TB, van der Zwaag AM, Schuurmans MJ. Leadership mentoring in nursing research, career development and scholarly productivity: a systematic review. Int J Nurs Stud. 2017;75:21–34.
4. Haines ST. The mentor-protégé relationship. Am J Pharm Educ. 2003;67(3):82.
5. Horner DK. Mentoring: positively influencing job satisfaction and retention of new hire nurse practitioners. Plast Surg Nurs. 2017;37(1):7–22.
6. Jnah AJ, Robinson CB. Mentoring and self-efficacy: implications for the neonatal nurse practitioner workforce. Adv Neonatal Care. 2015;15(5):E3–E11.
7. Sambunjak D, Straus SE, Marušić A. Mentoring in academic medicine: a systematic review. JAMA. 2006;296(9):1103–15.
8. Stamm M, Buddeberg-Fischer B. The impact of mentoring during postgraduate training on doctors' career success. Med Educ. 2011;45(5):488–96.
9. Brunt BA, Russell J. Nursing professional development standards. In: StatPearls [internet]. Treasure Island: StatPearls Publishing. 2021. https://www.ncbi.nlm.nih.gov/books/NBK534784/. Accessed 30 Oct 2021.
10. Straus SE, Johnson MO, Marquez C, Feldman MD. Characteristics of successful and failed mentoring relationships: a qualitative study across two academic health centers. Acad Med. 2013;88(1):82–9.
11. Carey E, Weissman D. Understanding and finding mentorship: a review for junior faculty. J Palliat Med. 2010;13(11):1373–9.
12. Smesny AL, Williams JS, Brazeau GA, et al. Barriers to scholarship in dentistry, medicine, nursing, and pharmacy practice faculty. Am J Pharm Educ. 2007;71(5):91.
13. Coleman VH, Power ML, Williams S, Carpentieri A, Schulkin J. Continuing professional development: racial and gender differences in obstetrics and gynecology residents' perceptions of mentoring. J Contin Educ Heal Prof. 2005;25(4):268–77.
14. Murphy M, Record H, Callander JK, Dohan D, Grandis JR. Mentoring relationships and gender inequities in academic medicine: findings from a multi-institutional qualitative study. Acad Med. 2022;97(1):136–42.
15. Byerley JS. Mentoring in the era of #MeToo. JAMA. 2020;323(17):1714–5.
16. Beech B, Calles-Escandon J, Hairston KG, et al. Mentoring programs for underrepresented minority faculty in academic medical centers: a systematic review of the literature. Acad Med. 2013;88(4):541–9.

17. Fang D, Moy E, Colburn L, Hurley J. Racial and ethnic disparities in faculty promotion in academic medicine. JAMA. 2000;284(9):1085–92.
18. Palepu A, Carr PL, Friedman RH, et al. Minority faculty and academic rank in medicine. JAMA. 1998;280(9):767–71.
19. Carmel RG, Paul MW. Mentoring and coaching in academia: reflections on a mentoring/coaching relationship. Policy Futures Educ. 2015;13(4):479–91.
20. Gazelle G, Liebschutz JM, Riess H. Physician burnout: coaching a way out. J Gen Intern Med. 2015;30(4):508–13.
21. Huff J, Preston C, Goldring E. Implementation of a coaching program for school principals: evaluating coaches' strategies and the results. Educ Manag Admin Lead. 2013;41(4):504–26.
22. Pinaud IM. Values clarification for student coaching. 2018. https://coachcampus.com/coach-portfolios/research-papers/isabelmonreal-pinaud-values-clarification-for-student-career-coaching/. Accessed 1 Sept 2023.
23. Kashiwagi DT, Varkey P, Cook DA. Mentoring programs for physicians in academic medicine: a systematic review. Acad Med. 2013;88(7):1029–37.
24. Manuel SP, Poorsattar SP. Mentoring up: twelve tips for successfully employing a mentee-driven approach to mentoring relationships. Med Teach. 2021;43(4):384–7.
25. Geraci SA, Thigpen SC. A review of mentoring in academic medicine. Am J Med Sci. 2017;353(2):767–71.
26. Davis OC, Nakamura J. A proposed model for an optimal mentoring environment for medical residents: a literature review. Acad Med. 2010;85(6):1060–6.
27. Hayes EF. Factors that facilitate or hinder mentoring in the nurse practitioner preceptor/student relationship. Clin Excell Nurse Pract. 2001;5(2):111–8.
28. Nick JM, Delahoyde TM, Del Prato D, et al. Best practices in academic mentoring: a model for excellence. Nurs Res Pract. 2012;2012:937906.
29. Zerzan JT, Hess R, Schur E, Phillips RS, Rigotti N. Making the most of mentors: a guide for mentees. Acad Med. 2009;84(1):140–4.
30. Thorndyke LE, Gusic ME, Milner RJ. Functional mentoring: a practical approach with multi-level outcomes. J Contin Educ Health Prof. 2008;28(3):157–64.
31. Berk RA, Berg J, Mortimer R, Walton-Moss B, Yeo TP. Measuring the effectiveness of faculty mentoring relationships. Acad Med. 2005;80(1):66–71.
32. DeMeyer FS, DeMeyer S. Mentoring the next generation of authors. Semin Oncol Nurs. 2018;34(4):338–53.
33. Pololi LH, Knight SM, Dennis K, Frankel RM. Helping medical school faculty realize their dreams: an innovative, collaborative mentoring program. Acad Med. 2002;77(5):377–84.
34. Henry-Noel N, Bishop M, Gwede CK, Petkova E, Szumacher E. Mentorship in medicine and other health professions. J Cancer Educ. 2019;34(4):629–37.
35. Hitchcock MA, Bland CJ, Hekelman FP, Blumenthal MG. Professional networks: the influence of colleagues on the academic success of faculty. Acad Med. 1995;70(12):1108–16.
36. Giancola JK, Whitman B, Wilmott RW. Establishing a mentoring culture within the department: the role of the chair. J Pediatr. 2020;225:4–7.e3.
37. Maisel NC, Halvorson MA, Finney JW, et al. Institutional incentives for mentoring at the U.S. Department of Veterans Affairs and universities: associations with mentors' perceptions and time spent mentoring. Acad Med. 2017;92(4):521–7.
38. Cataldi ML, Kelly-Hedrick M, Nanavati J, Chisolm MS, Anne LW. Post-residency medical education fellowships: a scoping review. Med Educ Online. 2021;26(1):1920084.
39. Tekian A, Harris I. Preparing health professions education leaders worldwide: a description of masters-level programs. Med Teach. 2012;34(1):52–8.

Chapter 17
Leadership and Health Scholars

Richard G. Milter and Kathleen M. White

17.1 Introduction

*Leadership is a function of knowing yourself, having a **vision** that is well communicated, **building trust** among colleagues, and **taking effective action** to realize your own leadership potential*—Warren Bennis

In today's competitive world, the challenge is to develop and exhibit leadership skills crucial for both personal and professional environments. Leadership is often defined as influence, which is the art of influencing people so that they will willingly and enthusiastically move toward the achievement of group goals. A leader is one who motivates followers toward some future direction and vision. This chapter describes the meaning of leadership through a discussion of the characteristics and qualities of effective leaders necessary to lead in our current and future dynamic work settings.

17.2 Visionary

Leadership for today's work requires a person who has vision, is a risk taker, and is not afraid to face change with fortitude. Goleman [1] described visionary leaders as those who … "articulate where the group is going, but not how it will get

R. G. Milter (✉)
The Johns Hopkins Carey Business School, Baltimore, MD, USA
e-mail: milter@jhu.edu

K. M. White
Johns Hopkins University School of Nursing, Johns Hopkins University School of Education, Baltimore, MD, USA
e-mail: kwhite2@jhu.edu

A. S. Fitzgerald, G. Bosch (eds.), *Education Scholarship in Healthcare*,
https://doi.org/10.1007/978-3-031-38534-6_17

there—setting people free to innovate, experiment, take calculated risks." Visionary leaders see potential and opportunity and often see what no one else does. They think about and plan for the future with innovation and creativity. The visionary leader is able to help others see and understand this vision and their role in achieving that vision for the future. They are inspirational and able to motivate others to turn the vision into a course of action and move others forward.

Today's evolving workplace is critically referred to as a VUCA environment, a work environment that displays unending volatility, uncertainty, complexity, and ambiguity [2]. This term was coined at the end of the Cold War by the US military and was meant to describe the fog of war where fighting capabilities are uncertain due to the unclear situations and rapidly changing conditions. Today, the volatility derives from the unprecedented change being experienced, uncertainty from the unpredictability about the future, complexity because of increasing interconnectedness and relatedness, and ambiguity from the world's continued confusion and chaos that affects our workplaces. This is the environment and the challenge that our leaders face today. We need strong visionary leaders who can lead through the fog, setting a positive course and realistic direction for today and into the future. This visionary leader will communicate and support workers through change and guide their organization to success.

17.3 Bravery

Leaders have long sought to hang tough onto their foundational values. And yet, leadership means helping others learn to value movement into the future which can be volatile, uncertain, complex, and ambiguous [2]. As scholar leaders in healthcare today, it is more important than ever to take a brave stance in reimagining what healthcare could look like and how new systems of delivery might more appropriately deliver benefits to global health. Brené Brown, globally recognized for her research on courage and leadership, defines a leader as "anyone who takes responsibility for finding the potential in people and processes, and who has the courage to develop that potential" ([3]: 4).

Brave leaders are not steely combative warriors but rather individuals who have learned how to "rumble with vulnerability" and possess a "grounded confidence" with their ability to remain curious in the face of uncertainty ([3]: 171). Bravery, as we refer to it here, is not about attempting to control everything but continuing to address uncertain and ambiguous situations with appreciative inquiry. The practice of asking generative questions to develop greater understanding is key to taking a brave stance as a leader. The focus of appreciative inquiry, which was born out of work in healthcare settings, is not on fixing problems by finding and placing blame. This practice is one of inviting others to chime in on what is working and use it to generate the next steps to be taken to address the concern [4]. The openness and ability to generate conversations among a diverse set of individuals require commitment and tenacity only displayed by the bravest of leaders.

Bravery for health scholars is steeped in the caring orientation that is foundational for health professions. Leaders who lose sight of this orientation can become mired in behavior that appears self-serving and presents as toxic for others. Brave leaders in the health sciences are those who protect the caring orientation and continually work to better understand the needs of those being served and those providing service.

17.4 Integrity

Integrity, known as the quality of being honest and having unshakable moral principles, is essential for trust in the leader-employee relationship. The foundation of integrity is consistent actions and strong values that are exhibited by people who do the right thing, even when no one is looking, and especially when it is difficult to do so.

In 2016, Forbes studied the leadership attributes among workers and chief financial officers (CFOs) to test their value of the following characteristics: accessibility, collaborative mindset, competitiveness, decisiveness, fairness, integrity, strategic mindset, and transparency. Both groups placed integrity at the top of the list, and 75% of workers ranked integrity as the most valued leadership characteristic as did 46% of CFOs. In addition, both groups ranked fairness as the second-highest valued characteristic by 58% of workers and 45% of CFOs. After those two related characteristics, the order of importance differed between the groups. Employees associate integrity with reliability, honesty, fairness, respectfulness, and having good intentions as opposed to selfish motives. Integrity engenders trust and respect from followers and is a quality that they use to measure leader competence. A leader with integrity builds trust and credibility, uses courage to face the challenges ahead, and inspires workers to commit to doing their best to achieve success. Leading with integrity means the leader holds themselves accountable as well as their colleagues and workers and admits vulnerability when things go wrong.

As a leader, your integrity modeled for your direct reports sets workplace expectations. Engaging in and supporting positive workplace behaviors, acting responsibly through fair and transparent decision-making, and upholding workplace values create a healthy work environment for everyone.

17.5 Magnanimity

Merriam-Webster defines magnanimity as a quality of possessing "loftiness of spirit enabling one to bear trouble calmly, to disdain meanness and pettiness, and to display a noble generosity." Magnanimity is a foundational element of leadership. It is a virtue that can be developed, refined, and expanded via practice and is a necessary element of leadership to build trust [5, 6]. The trust platform must be built on truth, not lies. Leaders displaying magnanimity typically also demonstrate genuine humility that engenders complementary qualities of self-control, courage, justice, and prudence. Only in this way can leaders promote a vision that is meaningful, bold, exciting, and realistic enough for others to join in the process of making that vision real.

Health scholars today are challenged by inept government and corporate leaders who have sought to politicize everything from human equity to public health. It is time for these leaders to work together in establishing evidence-based decisions that lead toward higher levels of leadership for all involved in maintaining and enriching the lives of others. But such collaborative approaches will not happen in the present milieu of political logjams. It is contingent upon health scholars to take up the challenge to serve the populations in their care.

Serving those who need care is in the very nature of what health scholars should keep front and center on their agendas. This suggests that health scholars are best able to solidify a trust relationship based upon full transparency of the methods used and results achieved by their investigations. Evidence-based research has long been the battle cry for health scholars. It is now time to consistently incorporate full evidence without the exclusion of facts that do not fully align with our hypotheses.

17.6 Creativity

Leadership is all about movement toward meaningful change. Creativity is "taking a proactive approach toward the production of novel or useful ideas that address a predicament or opportunity" [7]. Creative leadership is, therefore, a requirement for leading in any discipline, industry, or organization. It is especially necessary within the healthcare industry, which is experiencing a tremendous change in the educational landscape as well as in its delivery and financial systems. For the health scholar and leader, it is particularly important to be able to take a fresh and unobstructed view toward an evidence-based approach to future scenarios that would best serve the public good.

Traditions from basic to applied research and systematic reviews are all grounded in an acceptance of the scientific method, which stipulates that questions must drive exploration to test hypotheses and generate meaningful insights toward greater understanding. It is this type of inquisitiveness that Abraham Lincoln solicited in his remark that "the dogmas of the quiet past will not work in the turbulent future; as our cause is new so must we think and act anew." It is leader creativity that Albert Einstein elicited when he explained that no problem can be solved by the same consciousness that created it.

When she described the value of chaos theory leading to an awakening of creativity, Margaret Wheatley challenged us to take advantage of disruptive occurrences and embrace the dissipative activity as an opportunity for change [8]. For many scholar leaders in the healthcare industry, this concept is reminiscent of the work of Prigogine [9] and others who synthesize knowledge to connect systems from one discipline to applications across other domains. The ability to think creatively is what will more aptly lead scholarly research to impactful and sometimes groundbreaking new concepts and practices. Health scholar leaders are, thus, encouraged to see current disruptive practices in the healthcare industry as opportunities to expand their creative thinking and seek meaningful change.

17.7 Teaming

Leadership is not a destination but a journey. It is not a position but a practice. It is not a solitary endeavor but requires the full-hearted participation of others. Prior to the 1970s, most writers in the field of organizational behavior and organization design targeted the role of management. In fact, most of the management theories of the past century dealt with how to structure and form organizations for the highest efficiencies [10]. Little attention was paid to other things. One of the greatest known management theorists early in the last century, Frederick W. Taylor, advised that efficiency came from knowing exactly what you want men to do ... seeing that they do it in the best and cheapest way. Moving from Taylor to Max Weber to Henri Fayol to Henry Ford, the focus of their efforts was primarily on "getting the most out of the workforce" and little else. Henry Ford is said to have once proclaimed in frustration, "all I wanted was a pair of hands, and I got a brain as well."

As we moved from the industrial revolution where production efficiency was the primary goal to the knowledge economy where creativity reigns supreme, we have also seen the advantages of an evolution of language. It was not until late in the last century that the word group was in many instances replaced with the word team when considering organizational units. Up until that time, organizations were run by managers who in some cases incorporated group projects. Although these two words are often used interchangeably, there is a clear distinction between a group and a team. One delineation is that groups are a collection of individuals, each contributing their personal share to the end goal, which is established by a manager who is typically outside the group. A team, on the other hand, is comprised of individuals who together establish the procedures and formulations for how to best achieve the agreed-upon goals.

The concept of teaming has made clear paths in the healthcare industry in recognition of the heightened performance quality that can be achieved with a fully functioning team. Teaming has demonstrated value from the conference rooms to the breakrooms, from the executive level (C-suite) to the operating room, and from the emergency department to the registered dietician. Leaders in the healthcare industry are challenged to position teams and groups in their respective places and know when to transition from one to the other.

Health scholar leaders also need to establish a foundation of trust that will engender team members to trust each other, participate in meaningful conflict conversations, achieve consensual commitment to their goals, and hold each other accountable as they work to achieve results [11]. Leaders should seek to create a culture of psychological safety where members feel safe to take risks and make mistakes without fear of penalty or humiliation [12].

17.8 Servant

The term servant leader was first introduced by Robert Greenleaf in his 1970 essay that described a style of leadership as "The servant-leader [who] is servant first … begins with a natural feeling that one wants to serve, to serve first." The servant leader puts the needs of others first to empower them to be their best. In servant leadership, the leader puts the needs of followers first to empower them to be their best and ensures that they are growing in all areas of knowledge and development. This style of leadership has become popular in many of today's leading companies, such as Google and Southwest Airlines, whose leaders focus on their employees and increase employee satisfaction, growth, and productivity. The servant leader is known to have characteristics of good listening, empathy, healing, self-awareness, persuasive encouragement, visionary, foresight, stewardship, commitment, and a focus on building community.

This value of service for leaders has gained momentum as we move through the experience of dealing with global pandemics and more fully incorporating processes for expanding diversity, equity, inclusion, and belonging into our organizational culture. It was fairly obvious during the initial outbreak of COVID-19 who were the leaders that made the greatest impact on our future. They were not the leaders who ignored the science or looked for shortcuts to placate or dismiss the deadly virus. On the contrary, the leaders who stepped up and provided the pathways for dealing with the life-changing pandemic were those who demonstrated the aforementioned characteristics and placed the needs of many above their personal ambitions. It is that kind of leadership that most likely will stand the test of time as it demonstrates a supportive and encouraging role that is necessary as we meet the heightened demands ahead.

17.9 Listener

Listening, often referred to as soft leadership skill, is an important characteristic desired by all styles of leadership. Active listening, a hallmark of positive communication, is the foundation for the development of trust and respect between leaders and followers. Leaders who are engaged and actively listen to their workers show interest in those employees and create trustworthy relationships that produce loyalty.

Listening is a leadership responsibility that does not appear in the job description. Good listening skills in our digital era are fast becoming a lost art that requires leadership focus.

Even successful leaders will admit that listening can be a full-time job when you consider the VUCA environment of our current workplaces. Leaders who focus on listening to their employees are in a better position to lead through VUCA and to collaborate with an increasingly diverse and multigenerational workforce. An Interact/Harris Poll of 1000 US workers (2015) revealed that 91% of those employees identified "communication issues" with their bosses as a pain point [13].

Strong leadership requires full attention to each member of the team to show that you are listening, not just hearing their discussion, and that you understand and care about their thoughts. The leader's responsibility is to connect and engage with the team and show presence, attentiveness, and interest in their colleagues and staff. The leader creates a vision and sets purpose and goals but needs input from peers and workers about the means to those ends. Consider using this powerful listening strategy, and routinely ask for input from your colleagues and staff with the simple phrase, "What do you think?"

A discussion of listening would not be complete without a few words on emotional intelligence, the ability to be self-aware, understand, and appropriately regulate one's own emotions and emotional responses. The key to effective leadership is to be able to recognize, understand, and empathize with others through emotional intelligence. As you develop your leadership listening focus, ponder a quote from the Dalai Lama who said, *"When you speak, you repeat what you know. When you listen, you learn something new."* Listen to others and then show courage with your leadership.

17.10 Innovation

Although developing and engendering a creative mindset is important to leaders, it is not sufficient. Leaders also need to be skilled at leading innovation. A creative act is of little value unless it can lead to a product or service innovation. But leading innovation is more than saying, "I know the way ... follow me." Leading innovation is an all-inclusive activity of rallying everyone to take on the spirit and mindset of innovative practices. It is working to find the appropriate mix of unleashing some things and harnessing others. Activities to be unleashed include individual effort, support, learning and development, improvisation, patience, and a bottom-up orientation toward innovative practice. Things to be harnessed include collective effort, confrontation, performance, structure, urgency, and a top-down orientation.

A challenge for leaders is to be mindful and vigilant regarding the calibration and recalibration of actions to unleash or harness innovation across these somewhat paradoxical dimensions [14]. One of the core principles for leading innovation is to create and sustain a culture of learning where the permission to learn overrides the negative consequences of trial-and-error mistakes. This is perhaps most clearly illustrated by a sign in one of our biology labs that instructs the lab techs to "make new mistakes today." The emphasis is on stretching our thinking and expanding our boundaries so that new pathways can be discovered or designed. Leaders are people who, with creative agility, can encourage others to join in the pursuit of purposeful and commensurate adaptation in confronting vital challenges in need of change.

Health scholar leaders must be able to communicate and extend their personal commitment to impact the future of health science and health systems to others both inside and external to their sphere of basic science. Discovery research provides health scholars an opportunity to push against previously accepted boundaries. Health scholar leaders are challenged to help others see the value of discovery and help them to connect the dots for a brighter and more realistic view of the future.

17.11 Resilience

Change is perhaps the most important outcome of genuine leadership. But it is not change directed by a leader that matters. What matters most is change resulting from the collective genius of the entire organization. Leaders are those individuals who value contributions from diverse perspectives and have the courage to be open to various means and ways to meet current and future challenges. Not only do resilient leaders value diversity, but they also seek it out via a foundation of trust that is generated by sharing their personal vulnerabilities. Leaders are confident in who they are and are open about things they do well and things they do not do well. This openness to others is a demonstration of vulnerability that can be used as a model for others to share things about challenges they face.

Vulnerability-based leadership can only be exhibited when leaders drop their armor and become daring. Armored leadership is characterized as driving perfectionism and fostering fear of failure, being a knower and being right, and leading from hurt. Daring leadership, on the other hand, is characterized as modeling and encouraging healthy striving, empathy, and self-compassion; being a learner and getting it right; and leading from heart [3]. It takes genuine courage to practice daring leadership over armored leadership. It is simply easier to do what you want, put on our armor, and expect others to follow. This fear-mongering approach to leadership is anything but resilient as it promotes a false sense of security as followers are either kept in the dark or even misled by unclear or untrue proclamations.

Rather than hedging their actions on fantasy and misinformation, resilient leaders encourage others to perform beyond perceived limits and extend capabilities to address the most difficult crises. According to George Everly, a pioneer in the field of human resilience, there are six key principles of resilient leadership: (1) following the moral compass of integrity; (2) using the power of communication, persuasion, and inspiration; (3) demonstrating vision and optimism; (4) taking responsibility for one's actions and having perseverance; (5) building a resilient culture; and (6) developing stress management as a competitive advantage [15]. This final principle has been termed psychological body armor when used to protect yourself and behavioral body armor when a leader uses it to help protect others.

Scholar leaders in healthcare should be particularly attuned to both types of armor as they support the work of others to cure illness, promote wellness, and protect against disease. These health scholar leaders should work toward personal health and safety as they continue to help others do the same. They might be best able to serve others by donning psychological body armor and taking actions to protect others from being left behind, overtrodden, ignored, or simply cast aside. As we face challenging times, it is our leaders who act with resilience who can help us to shape a better future. Health scholar leaders should see it as their duty to help shape the future of healthcare and protect the resilience of those in their care.

17.12 Conclusions: Leadership for the Future

The challenge for the health scholar leader of the future is to ask what makes a good leader and is there a preferred style of leadership. There is no simple answer to that question, and as you can see from reading this chapter, we targeted key characteristics and qualities for leadership. The development of strong leadership depends on your ability to learn and use different leadership styles at different times in different situations. We started with the discussion of the visionary leader and discussed other qualities of leadership, choosing to end with innovation and resilience as important strengths in any leadership situation. The challenge is yours to discover and build

Table 17.1 Leadership qualities and skills for implementation

Leader qualities	Key skills for implementation by health scholar leaders		
Visionary	Set direction	Take risk	Inspiration and motivation
Bravery	Ask generative questions	Target what is working	Focus on serving and served
Integrity	Honesty, trust, and respect	Accountability and vulnerability	Role model
Magnanimity	Display a noble generosity	Seek truth and refute lies	Display noble generosity
Creativity	Take fresh and unobstructed view	See disruptive occurrences as opportunity for change	Connect learnings across disciplines and industries
Teaming	Need full-hearted participation of all	Allow teams to self-direct	Engender trust
Servant	Servant first	Empower others	Ensure growth and development
Listener	Active engagement	Seek understanding and show caring	Exhibit emotional intelligence
Innovation	Rally others to take on the spirit	Remain mindful and vigilant	Create and sustain a culture of learning
Resilience	Recognize collective genius and diversity	Protect self with psychological body armor	Seek out potential in others and protect them with behavioral body armor

your leadership for the complex and dynamic academic work environment you have chosen for yourself as a health scholar leader (Table 17.1).

17.13 Questions

Discussion
1. Which of the characteristics highlighted in this chapter do you find to be most connected to your work as a leader?

   (a) What steps would you initially take to further develop these leadership capabilities in your organization?

2. Consider a leader you admire. What are the key characteristics that come to mind? How do the characteristics of your most admired leader compare to the capabilities illustrated in this chapter?

Activities
1. Take each of the capabilities listed in the table in this chapter and provide one or two action steps you could take to incorporate the capability more fully in your leadership activity.
2. For each of the capabilities illustrated in this chapter, provide a leader you believe best demonstrates that capability.

References

1. Goleman D. What makes a leader? Harv Bus Rev. 1998;76:93–102.
2. Bennett N, Lemoine GJ. What VUCA really means for you. Harv Bus Rev. 2014;92(1/2).
3. Brown B. Dare to Lead. London: Vermilion Press; 2018.
4. Cooperrider DL, Whitney D. Appreciative inquiry: a positive revolution in change. San Francisco: Berrett-Koehler Publishers; 2005.
5. Covey SM. The SPEED of trust: the one thing that changes everything. 2018.
6. Havard A. Virtuous leadership: an agenda for personal excellence. Scepter. 2007.
7. Puccio G, Mance M, Murdock M. Creative leadership: skills that drive change. Thousand Oaks: SAGE Publications; 2011.
8. Wheatley M. Leadership and the new science. Oakland: Berrett-Koehler; 2006.
9. Prigogine I. The end of certainty: time, chaos, and the new laws of nature. New York: The Free Press; 1998.
10. Hamel G. The future of management. Boston: Harvard Business School Press; 2007.
11. Lencioni P. The advantage. San Francisco: Jossey-Bass; 2012.
12. Edmondson AC. Teaming: how organizations learn, innovate, and compete in the knowledge economy. San Francisco: Jossey-Bass; 2012.
13. Solomon L. The top complaints from employees about their leaders. Harv Bus Rev. 2015;93(5/6).

14. Hill LA, Brandeau G, Truelove E, Lineback K. Collective genius: the art and practice of leading innovation. Boston: Harvard Business Review Press; 2014.
15. Everly GS Jr, Stouse DA, Everly GS III. The secrets of resilient leadership. New York: DiaMedica Publishing; 2010.

Part VI
More Depth for the Enthusiast

Chapter 18
Appendix

April S. Fitzgerald, Sharon K. Park, Khanh-Van Le-Bucklin, Julie Youm, and Ahmed Ibrahim

18.1 Introduction

In this Appendix, we have added additional material beyond what is offered in the chapters for readers wanting additional depth.

18.2 Case Examples Demonstrating Elements of Glassick's Criteria

Sharon K. Park Khanh-Van Le-Bucklin, and Julie Youm

The following case examples are presented to illustrate the application of Glassick's criteria to different research scenarios:

A. S. Fitzgerald (✉)
Division of General Internal Medicine, Department of Medicine, Johns Hopkins University School of Medicine, Baltimore, MD, USA
e-mail: afitzg10@jhmi.edu

S. K. Park
School of Pharmacy, Notre Dame of Maryland University, Baltimore, MD, USA
e-mail: spark@ndm.edu

K.-V. Le-Bucklin · J. Youm
University of California, Irvine School of Medicine, Irvine, CA, USA
e-mail: klebuckl@uci.edu; jyoum@uci.edu

A. Ibrahim
Johns Hopkins University School of Education, Baltimore, MD, USA
e-mail: aibrahim@jhu.edu

A. S. Fitzgerald, G. Bosch (eds.), *Education Scholarship in Healthcare*, https://doi.org/10.1007/978-3-031-38534-6_18

18.2.1 Case 1: Overall Research (Glassick's Criteria 1–6)

LJ is a final-year fellow who is highly interested in pursuing a career as a physician educator. She recently designed and implemented an orientation curriculum for new fellows based on her own experience as a fellow. This training included a shadowing session with a senior fellow, strategies for teaching medical students and residents, and advice on how to approach new consults.

LJ is interested in disseminating her work and consults with an education dean to discuss how best to move forward. In consideration of Glassick's criteria, she is asked the following questions:

1. What is the purpose of the orientation curriculum? Why is this new curriculum necessary? (Standard 1)
2. What were the curriculum's learning objectives? (Standard 1) How do you define success or benefit from the curriculum?
3. How is this curriculum unique from other fellowship orientation training described in the literature? What were the benefits to the internal and external stakeholders? (Standards 1 and 2)
4. Who is involved in the development, implementation, assessment, data collection, and analysis? Are there adequate support and mentors as resources to complete the project successfully? (Standard 2)
5. What are the methods used to measure desired outcomes? (Standard 3)
6. What are the results? How would they be analyzed? (Standard 4)
7. How are the results presented? Are they presented based on the appropriate medium, audience, length, and depth? Are the results presented in a clear and relevant way? (Standards 4 and 5)
8. What are the goals for dissemination? What would be the most effective or efficient method of dissemination? Are there resources to ensure these plans? (Standard 5)
9. What does the data inform about the orientation curriculum? What did she learn from the first implementation that she might apply to future course offerings? (Standard 6)

LJ shares that she did not have formal learning objectives and that the curriculum was based on gaps in knowledge and skills that she recalled having as a new fellow. She had not conducted a literature review and thus was unable to describe how the curriculum was unique from orientations for fellows in other programs at her medical school or at other institutions. The curriculum had been designed and implemented largely independently, and she had not developed any associated learner assessments or program evaluations.

In discussion with LJ, she is commended for her enthusiasm for education and a curriculum that was designed with the intention of making the transition into fellowship easier for her more junior colleagues. While LJ would have benefited from mentorship early in her design of the curriculum, she is encouraged to pursue her goal to ultimately disseminate her work. She is given the following advice based on Glassick's criteria:

1. Write in one or two sentences the purpose of the curriculum and the goals of the research study. (Standard 1)
2. For each session of the curriculum, develop associated learning objectives with clear and measurable outcomes. (Standard 1)
3. Conduct a literature review to understand what is being done at other institutions, ascertain how the training is unique, and/or how this adds to current literature on the subject. (Standards 1 and 2)
4. Find a faculty mentor who can work with her on developing research questions and methods of assessment. (Standard 2)
5. Develop and conduct assessments. (Standard 3)
6. Analyze results to address the research goals. (Standard 4)
7. Begin the dissemination process with a poster presentation at a medical education conference or specialty conference where there is a special call for trainee-authored posters. (Standard 5)
8. Include in the poster results, limitations, lessons learned, and next steps. (Standard 6)

LJ takes the advice above and develops goals and objectives. Given that participants had just completed the training, at the advice of her mentor, she conducts a retrospective pre-post survey as well as a qualitative analysis of feedback from participants. Her plan is to adjust and expand her assessment methods in future course offerings. She plans to develop a poster for presentation to disseminate her work.

18.2.2   Case 2: Lack of Clear and Achievable Goals (Glassick's Criteria 1)

HB is a third-year cardiology resident who is interested in pursuing education research before transitioning to a fellowship. He met with his attending to discuss his ideas around exploring the impact of wearable heart rate monitors on managing patients with arrhythmia or an irregular heartbeat. The attending encouraged HB to apply for department funds to purchase and distribute wearable heart rate monitors to the patients he treats. The department was interested in learning more about these new technologies and awarded him the funds for the study. HB recruits patients for his study by providing them a new wearable device and asking them to share daily electrocardiogram (ECG) readings with him via email. He conducts a physical exam and collects some demographic information from each patient at the start of the study, e.g., gender, age, race/ethnicity, height, weight, blood pressure, pulse rate, and respiration rate, along with responses to a survey about patients' interests and experiences with wearable devices. HB then collects ECGs from study participants over a period of a month. At the end of the month, patients were asked to come back for another physical exam, and vital sign data is collected again.

After the data collection period, HB prepared to analyze the ECGs he received and make some conclusions about the effectiveness of wearable heart rate monitors for this patient population. However, without a clearly defined research question, HB struggles with drawing any significant and meaningful conclusions from the wealth of data he has collected. His excitement to understand and evaluate a trending technology innovation in his field was not accompanied by a thoughtful and systematic approach to assess its efficacy. While the data could yield some exploratory findings, the lack of clear goals and research questions makes it difficult to determine if his research approach was adequate for any further conclusions or implications of his work.

18.2.3 Case 3: Lack of Thorough Preparation (Glassick's Criteria 2)

SY is a hospitalist in internal medicine and a new assistant professor at a school of medicine. She was provided with a $2000 stipend to be used toward her education research during her first 3 years in this position. For the past 2 years, she was busy establishing her practice and helping run the service with several new practice protocols. Since this is her last year to use the fund, she attempts to conduct an education research project that she feels could be performed with minimal effort. Recalling her own positive learning experiences with residents as a medical student, she decides that an easy hypothesis to confirm would be as follows: "Third-year medical students on the internal medicine clerkship learn better on teams with residents than without residents." SY selects summative clerkship exam scores as her only assessment method for comparing learning between the two groups because this data is readily available. She is surprised to find no significant difference in the mean exam scores of the groups and hastily concludes that students do not learn better on teams with residents.

It is not uncommon for an inexperienced clinician educator to jump right into an education research project with an assumption that the input (educational interventions) should clearly demonstrate an output (e.g., increased knowledge and skills). However, because education research deals mainly with people, their behaviors and attitudes, and various confounding variables (e.g., age, experience), thorough preparation and a potentially complex methodology beyond randomization and blinding are required to reach a successful research process. In addition, multiple levels of learning may need to be assessed to differentiate between control and study groups in education research studies. In this case, SY felt rushed to begin her research and use allocated funds before they expired; thus, there was a lack of time, effort, and resources fully engaged for her to adequately develop her study. It would be advised for SY to conduct a thorough review of existing scholarship, consult content and methodological experts, and write a research protocol with clear goals and assessment methods.

18.2.4 Case 4: Mismatched Evaluation and Outcomes (Glassick's Criteria 3)

JW is a nurse practitioner who teaches a Pediatric Advanced Life Support (PALS) course for nurses. She typically teaches a 2-day course that consists of 50% traditional lecture and 50% hands-on training using low-fidelity mannequins. Following the building of a simulation center, she decides to teach the course using assigned online videos followed by a full day of hands-on training using high-fidelity simulators. To test her hypothesis that a flipped classroom instructional design with high-fidelity simulation is more effective than lecture and low-fidelity simulation, she compares the multiple-choice exam performance of current students with those from past course administrations. She finds no difference in mean exam scores and concludes that high-fidelity simulation is not more effective than low-fidelity simulation.

In this case, the researcher fails to clearly define the intended outcome in determining "effectiveness." While there appears to be no short-term difference in terms of performance on a knowledge-based multiple-choice assessment, a more salient evaluation of the curriculum might have been a delayed workplace-based knowledge and skill assessment since the intention of PALS training is to prepare nurses to manage real-world cardiopulmonary code situations. A delayed workplace-based mock code assessment might have served as a superior method of evaluation, with effectiveness defined as improvement in students' workplace performance.

18.2.5 Case 4: "So What?" Lack of Meaningful Outcomes (Glassick's Criteria 4)

OC is a family medicine physician with an interest in narrative medicine and has designed an elective course to introduce students to the practice. Session activities for the course included reading and analyzing poems and short stories, as well as engaging in creative writing. OC's hypothesis was that students will develop greater empathy for patients following the course. To assess whether students are more empathetic, OC had the students self-assess on a 5-point Likert scale their level of agreement with the statement "I feel empathy towards my patients." He conducted this assessment at the beginning and the end of the course. In analyzing the results, he found a significant difference between pre/post-course results and concluded that the course had improved students' empathy toward patients.

There are three potential issues with this study's outcomes. First, OC's method of assessment may not have been appropriate to adequately measure a meaningful difference in student empathy development. Other assessments he could have considered include a retrospective pre-post attitudinal survey or a validated empathy assessment instrument. A literature review of empathy assessment methods would have uncovered a number of ways to approach answering the research question. Implementing a combination of these methods may have produced more reliable and robust results. Second, the students may have been working and interacting with patients during the elective course, which could contribute to improving their empathy. This type of confounding factor is commonly encountered in health professions education where the outcome may not be due to a contribution of the intended intervention alone. In this case, having a comparison group of students who did not take the course and conducting a comparative analysis would be appropriate. Third, OC failed to provide an important connection between students' empathy development and its translation to patient care. Students "feeling empathy" may not actually present as empathetic care for patients. This is another reason why using a validated survey is necessary to demonstrate that perception leads to action. In addition to researching the body of published work on the subject matter, other approaches in selecting evaluation methods include consultation with a mentor, statistician, or expert in the field of narrative medicine.

18.2.6　Case 5: Underselling One's Hard Work (Glassick's Criteria 5)

TG is a clinical pharmacist who also serves as the course director for a first-year pharmacology course. She is interested in studying whether gamification has a positive effect on student retention of course material. To test her hypothesis that gamification is more effective than traditional lecture in terms of content retention, she employed a Jeopardy-style game for her pre-final course review. She spent several weeks developing games for the five most difficult pharmacotherapeutic topics she teaches including antimicrobials, cardiovascular drugs, and intravenous drug dosing. TG then compared the final exam performance of the current cohort of students with those who received a traditional PowerPoint lecture review session in prior years. She found no significant difference in mean exam scores and concluded that gamification does not improve course material retention. Initially, she had intended to present this research and its results at her school's faculty summer retreat; however, given the negative outcomes, she decided to not present or publish her work.

Developing novel instructional strategies such as gaming involves a lot of effort, especially when the instruction covers a diverse and expansive number of content areas as in TG's case. The true value of TG's research may not necessarily be whether gaming made a difference in the one-time measurement of exam scores but rather if the students found learning through gaming more helpful and engaging and the instructor more motivated to teach the subject. Therefore, the development and implementation of the game-based instruction and assessment (the "how") as well as the student's perception and attitude toward learning the content (a higher engagement and interest in learning) should have been considered as the outcomes of this research. The rationale for incorporating gaming in instruction may also serve as an important catalyst for implementing this intervention for another year or with a different cohort of students to test the hypothesis again with a larger sample size.

18.3   Focusing on the Scoping Review

Ahmed Ibrahim

Scoping reviews have seen a noticeable increase in publishing. One reason might be that the methodological framework for completing such a review was published by Arksey and O'Malley [1] and by Levac et al. [2]. Another might be that scholars have found scoping reviews to be a convenient methodology that provides a good balance between effort and returns on investment. Conducting a scoping review does not require the same amount of effort and resources that a systematic review or meta-analysis requires, yet the review gives a useful quality appraisal, can answer important questions, and has the potential to be published in a reputable journal. Additionally, the learning curve is less steep for doing a scoping review compared with other types of reviews.

A scoping review serves the purpose of providing an initial portrait of the literature on a specific topic. Use a scoping review:

- If the topic is new, vague, or requires a better understanding.
- If a scholar is new to a topic, conducts a preliminary search, and does not find any significant research on a topic. The scoping review provides a systematic approach to survey a deeper dive to look for what has been published.
- If the literature is scant or scattered, the scoping review is ideal to bring together multiple sources into a coherent picture that provides a better understanding.

The Arksey and O'Malley [1] framework is widely cited and used by most scoping review studies. Building on their work, several enhancements and recommendations helped improve the scoping review methodology. Recently, Westphaln et al. [3] synthesized these enhancements and recommendations to provide us with the most up-to-date framework as outlined below.

Step 1: Specify the research question

The first step of conducting a scoping review is to articulate a specific research question. Formulating a good research question that can be used as the basis of a scoping review requires some time and effort to state it in an informative and useful manner.

Step 2: Identify relevant literature

Next, search through different sources such as library databases, specific journals (called hand-searching), websites, relevant organizations, and conferences. This step requires a good understanding of electronic databases. Academic institutions often have databases available to health scholars through their institutional library websites. It is recommended that health scholars use the institution's library portal to access databases and other resources since many databases require a subscription for access, and many institutions have paid access.

Step 3: Select studies

The search process in Step 2 might yield a large number of results, but not all of these results should be included in the review. Based on the exclusion criteria that are defined by the health scholar and team, some results can be eliminated.

Step 4: Collecting, mapping, and charting the data

Now the scoping review needs data synthesis and interpretation. A pilot of the data collection process with at least two team members before launching across the entire team is recommended. The data can then be analyzed quantitatively and qualitatively with a side-by-side comparison.

Step 5: Summarizing, synthesizing, and reporting the results

It is highly recommended to offer insights and identify gaps in addition to the summary, synthesis, and reporting. This allows the substantive, thorough, sophisticated, and meaningful literature review to act as a stepping stone for further research.

Step 6: Integrating expert consultation

In this final step, it is recommended to invite expert consultants to provide feedback, comment on results, and link these results to new research or historical context. While Arksey and O'Malley [1] suggested this step in their original framework as optional, other authors have considered this step essential.

18.4 History of Abstracts

Emily L. Jones

Since the first scientific article was published in France in 1665, the act of publication has been the predominant way to communicate the advancement of scientific work to others [6]. The first scientific journals were collections of letters, one of the main ways that scientists and scholars communicated with each other prior to the advent of journals [4]. The advent of journals meant that scientific discourse could happen outside private correspondence between the privileged class and in an arena with more access to the public.

The early consumers of scientific journals were mostly primarily upper-class men. These gentlemen scholars living through the Age of Enlightenment and the scientific advances of the Victorian era saw major advances in science and an explosion of related scientific discourse. Memberships in clubs such as the Royal Society of London swelled as did the number of and specialization of these scientific societies—some with the express purpose of publishing new journals or presenting papers in front of their memberships [7]. As more journals were published, it became more difficult for audiences to keep up with so much new scientific information.

This abundance of scholarship produced the need to be able to sort through information in an organized manner. The first scientific abstracts were not written by the author of the research, but by writers hired to summarize research for busy men of science, who did not have the time or more likely the inclination to go through every article being produced. In the early 1800s, the Royal Society used the word abstract to mean the summary—usually written by a secretary, rather than the author—of a paper that had been read at a scientific meeting.

As the speed at which research was undertaken increased, abstracts started to appear as a regular accompaniment to scientific papers in the 1930s. Having evolved from the letter format, most journals featured a format closer to a scientific report [9]. Much of what we now consider the process by which scientific experiments are conducted and disseminated comes from Louis Pasteur's work during this period.

In Louis Pasteur's book Etudes sur la Biere, he conscientiously describes each study he undertakes in such a descriptive manner that the work could be replicated. While he does not use the headings that now comprise the acronym IMRAD, Day [4] suggests that Pasteur invented the logical flow of content that we now know as this process. During the 50 years that followed Pasteur's work, some of the early twentieth century's biggest scientific advances such as the discovery of Salvarsan, penicillin, and sulfa drugs were published in papers that appear almost modern in their format [4].

In the scientific boom that followed the Cold War's space race in the late 1950s, the United States invested heavily in science, increasing the number of scientific publications that came from this funding exponentially. In order to sort through such an increased amount of submissions, journal editors became increasingly insistent on tightly written research papers that followed a logical progression through the scientific method [4]. In 1972, the IMRAD format was formally adopted as the standard for most scientific journals following the publication of the American National Standard for the preparation of scientific papers for written or oral presentation (ANSI Z39.16-1972). Structured abstracts became more common in medical journals during the 1990s. Nakayama (2005) [10] found that among the top 30 scientific medical journals, according to impact factors, just over 60% used the IMRAD structure for reporting their findings, while close to 40% used a different format.

While the number of scientific journals has grown to over 30,000 journals today, the growth rate has not been steady, rising and slowing in accordance with changing world politics and major advances in technology [8]. Between 1986 and 2013, academic journals grew at an average of 4.7% per year, roughly equal to the rate of growth between 1944 and 1978, an era often referred to in research on the history of scientific scholarship as the era of "Big Science" [5].

According to the 2018 STM Report, consumers of scientific content read on average 250 journal articles a year, a number that appears to be stabilizing after a decades-long increase. It is unclear if that is because the reader reaches saturation, but we do know that readers are spending an average of 30 min on each article, down from the 40–45 min readers spent on individual articles in the 1990s. Social media may also play a part in how researchers find articles as many scientists in the same or similar fields may be connected through social networking sites where they publicize their research as it comes out.

References

1. Arksey H, O'Malley L. Scoping studies: towards a methodological framework. Int J Social Res Methodol. 2005;8(1):19–32. https://doi.org/10.1080/1364557032000119616.
2. Levac D, Colquhoun H, O'Brien KK. Scoping studies: advancing the methodology. Implement Sci. 2010;5:1–9.
3. Westphaln KK, Regoeczi W, Masotya M, Vazquez-Westphaln B, Lounsbury K, McDavid L, Lee H, Johnson J, Ronis SD. From Arksey and O'Malley and beyond: customizations to enhance a team-based, mixed approach to scoping review methodology. MethodsX. 2021;8:101375. https://doi.org/10.1016/j.mex.2021.101375.
4. Day RA. The origins of the scientific paper: the IMRAD format. Am Med Writers Assoc J. 1989;4:16–8.
5. Gu X, Blackmore KL. Recent trends in academic journal growth. Scientometrics. 2016;108(2):693–716.
6. Jinha AE. Article 50 million: an estimate of the number of scholarly articles in existence. Learned Publishing. 2010;23(3):258–263.
7. Kronick DA. Medical "publishing societies" in eighteenth-century Britain. Bull Med Library Assoc. 1994;82(3):277–82.
8. Mabe M, Amin M. Growth dynamics of scholarly and scientific journals. Scientometrics. 2001;51(1):147–62.
9. Sollaci LB, Pereira MG. The introduction, methods, results, and discussion (IMRAD) structure: a fifty-year survey. J Med Library Assoc. 2004;92(3):364.
10. Nakayama T, Hirai N, Yamazaki S, Naito M. Adoption of structured abstracts by general medical journals and format for a structured abstract. J Med Library Assoc. 2005;93(2):237.

Correction to: Ethics and Research

Michael Malinowski and Michael F. Amendola

Correction to:
Chapter 8 in: A. S. Fitzgerald, G. Bosch (eds.),
Education Scholarship in Healthcare,
https://doi.org/10.1007/978-3-031-38534-6_8

The author's last name was misspelled as Malinkowski instead of Malinowski in the original version of Chapter 8. The error has been corrected in the revised publication.

The updated version of this chapter can be found at
https://doi.org/10.1007/978-3-031-38534-6_8

A. S. Fitzgerald, G. Bosch (eds.), *Education Scholarship in Healthcare*,
https://doi.org/10.1007/978-3-031-38534-6_19

Index